Critical Social Theory

in Public Administration

Richard C. Box

M.E.Sharpe
Armonk, New York
London, England

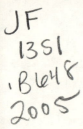
9515074

The author thanks Sage Publications, Inc. for permission to reprint material that first appeared in *American Review of Public Administration,* and *Administrative Theory & Praxis* for permission to reprint papers first published in that journal. Both publications allow authors to use their work in other venues.

Library of Congress Cataloging-in-Publication Data

Box, Richard C.
Critical social theory in public administration / by Richard C. Box.
  p. cm.
Includes bibliographical references and index.
ISBN 0-7656-1554-1 (cloth : alk. paper)
  1. Public administration—Philosophy. 2. Critical theory. 3. Frankfurt school of sociology. I. Title.

JF1351.B648 2004
351′.01′1—dc22   2004005154

Printed in the United States of America

The paper used in this publication meets the minimum requirements of American National Standard for Information Sciences Permanence of Paper for Printed Library Materials, ANSI Z 39.48-1984.

∞

BM (c) 10   9   8   7   6   5   4   3   2   1

Critical Social Theory

in Public Administration

Contents

Critical Social Theory

in Public Administration

Introduction

This book introduces a framework for the application of critical social theory in public administration. The goal is modest: to encourage awareness in public administration of societal conditions that tend to shape and constrain scholarship, teaching, practice, and social change. "Introduces" may not be the most appropriate word; there is nothing "new" about the contents of the framework and elements of it have been used for some time by public administration scholars and practitioners. It is not intended to compete as the latest fad management technique or innovation in public practice and it draws on materials that were written several decades ago.

Critical social theory was formulated by the Institute for Social Research (the "Frankfurt school") in 1937 as "critical theory of society" (Kellner, 2001, p. 9). With notable exceptions, it has been largely ignored in public administration, a field in which people concentrate on micro implementation rather than macro societal context and often avoid questioning oppressive or inequitable structures and practices. A central assumption of this book is that this is a good time in public administration to reflect upon our relationship to society, with attention to the desire of some scholars and practitioners to engage in thought and action designed to create constructive social change. The evidence for this assumption surrounds us in news of inequity, inequality, extreme concentration of wealth and power, pointless and damaging war and violence, and environmental destruction on a massive scale.

In broadest outline, critical social theory may be thought of as a vestige of utopian hopes for an alternative future. Following what he takes to be

Frederic Jameson's characterization of "postmodernism as the cultural logic of late capitalism, or capitalism in its phase of global hegemony" (Booker, 2002, p. 4), M. Keith Booker argues that the beginnings of postmodernism in the 1950s corresponded with the "ultimate collapse of the American utopian imagination" (p. 10). Caught in a "double bind of alienation and routinization," Americans "were terrified of being different, of not living up to the images of normality constantly beamed into the new television sets in their suburban living rooms," and yet:

> they were terrified of losing their individuality altogether, thus joining the series of anonymous and interchangeable cogs that made up the gears of the corporate machine. Meanwhile, there were lurking and potentially ominous reminders that not all Americans were so affluent, not to mention the vast majority of the population of the rest of the world. Thus, white, middle-class Americans came increasingly, in the long 1950s, to think of their lives as an island of prosperity and tranquillity surrounded by a threatening sea of poverty and turmoil, somewhat in the mode of those bands of pioneers who had long circled their wagons to fight off savage Indian attacks on American movie screens. (pp. 9–10)

For Booker (2001, pp. 11–15; 2002, pp. 7–8), this was the beginning of the end of serious attempts to conceptualize alternatives to late capitalism, despite critique of societal conditions by authors such as David Reisman (*The Lonely Crowd*, 1950), William Whyte (*The Organization Man*, 1956), and C. Wright Mills (*The Power Elite*, 1956), and the bubbling up of radical thought during the 1960s. Though he notes that postmodernism can be a source of critique and resistance to the dominant society, Booker (2002, p. 195) finds that "this anxious strain of postmodernism poses no real challenge to the hegemony of late capitalism, partly because of the ongoing absence of any effective utopian alternative." Theresa Ebert (1996, p. 148) is more optimistic, hoping to inject a materialist, economic critique of ideology and institutions into cultural postmodernism, in part by intervening "in the patriarchal capitalist knowledge industry." This will be difficult, since contemporary conditions are not friendly to critique of the status quo and discussion of alternatives within a global capitalist or postmodern society.

Given the difficulty of crafting large-scale interventions to counter effects of the current organization of society, the model of study and practice outlined here is a process, not an explicit blueprint for societal and organizational outcomes, though it includes broad normative description of an alternative future. The critical framework includes recognition of the tendency for late capitalist society to organize in ways that inhibit individual

and social development and a process for working toward local melioration. It does not assume the only path to change is radical, wholesale aban-
donment of current structures and practices. Instead, it acknowledges
individual and group resistance to damaging institutions and practices as a
valid way forward. On the theoretical level, Brian Fay (1987, p. 212) described a revitalized critical social science consisting of theories that are
"self-consciously local, particular, situated, experimental, and physical."
Exactly how theory building and application will occur in each setting or
issue circumstance will be decided by the people involved in specific times
and places.

There may be times when people are especially receptive to critical analysis of society because of current events. This is probably such a time, one in
which the normative ends and operating procedures of government push
the limits of what is considered appropriate. It is possible that in a few
years the current aggressive, poorly informed, destructive approach to people
and the environment demonstrated by neoliberal capitalist society may have
softened. However, the economic and institutional structures and practices
that support current conditions have existed for some time and will no doubt
continue into the foreseeable future. Perversely, it is fortunate for the purposes of critical analysis that the present state of affairs makes these matters particularly transparent, but this does not necessarily mean the
underlying structures and practices will change significantly if there are
different people in power who are more adept at obscuring them.

A Particular Form of Critical Social Theory

Today, many people think of critical theory as the same thing as the work of
Jürgen Habermas. As important as Habermas is to contemporary social science, some scholars regard his current writing as no longer especially critical, but rather reformist within the mainstream of political and philosophical
thought. A distinction often made between Habermas and his predecessors
in the Frankfurt school, including Herbert Marcuse, is his use of the dimension of intersubjective communication, thus decentering the subject and
acknowledging the socially constructed nature of human perception. However, Karl Marx (in Tucker, 1972, p. 223) recognized that humans are social creatures, and so did the first generation of Frankfurt theorists. The fact
that part of our understanding of social meaning is constructed inter-
subjectively does not negate individual values and intent. These are created
within a social milieu, but their character in each individual is unique.
Human behavior in intersubjective discourse settings is often a small part

of the overall process of decision making on public matters. Even if it were possible to create "ideal" discourse conditions in which differences in power and position were rendered inoperative, and even if it were possible to reach a noncoercive, democratic consensus on divisive, contentious issues (both heroic assumptions), discourse alone would seldom determine the course of events.

Critical social theory comes in several forms, but the one used here is the work of Herbert Marcuse. Often dismissed as too radical or out of date, Marcuse's thought frequently parallels contemporary thinking about ways to humanize organizations, interpersonal relations, governmental operations, and international affairs. It is the focus of this book because I have found it to be especially useful for understanding concrete, immediate matters of public practice, phenomena such as the politics-administration relationship and the penetration of economistic concepts into public governance.

As a practitioner in local government, I thought governmental systems to be biased against citizen awareness and ease of involvement, in favor of the interests of people with power and money who used government for personal financial benefit. Laws, policies, procedures, bureaucratic account-ability, and decision-making methods such as "public hearings" diminished citizen access and the possibility of considering a future with broader collective benefits. It was not that citizens in general were breathlessly awaiting the opportunity to spend time learning about complex public matters and discussing them with others. However, some people will do so, to the benefit of the human and physical world, given access to appropriate knowledge and the opportunity to use it.

This sense of lost opportunity in the current situation does not assume a unitary interest among the public or within the political and economic elite, nor a divergence of interests between political/economic decision makers and the broader community. Critical social theory assumes that the competitive, acquisitive nature of liberal-capitalist society is such that patterns of domination and repression will be present in some form in most settings, but the character of interests and purposes in a given place and time (whether the scale is global, national, regional, or local) can only be understood in that particular context. It also should be recognized that the nature of citizen access and opportunity varies from place to place and time to time. In some places and at some times, structures and practices have been changed so that the balance between the market imperative and the possibilities for self-governance has shifted significantly. However, where public inquiry and discourse is constrained, outcomes are relatively predictable and serve a narrow set of preferences.

Marcuse's work assists in understanding such situations because it offers a comprehensive view of the interactions among political and economic systems, technology, the natural environment, and human motivation. One reason he is often dismissed as a theorist is that people have not read the full body of his writing, which reaches from the 1930s to the 1970s. Instead, often only one work is discussed, usually *One-Dimensional Man*, and then in lopsided caricature. This is sloppy scholarship and it misses a rich, complex, and quite accessible body of material that forms a strikingly thorough and pertinent conceptual context for our times. (Perspective on the full range of Marcuse's thought has recently been expanded by release of books of his collected papers, edited by Douglas Kellner.) In addition to the problem of errors due to lack of knowledge, there is also the matter of Marcuse's lack of fit with current philosophical sensibilities. Douglas Kellner (1998, p. xiii) describes Marcuse at the peak of scholarly and public awareness of his ideas:

> During the late 1960s and 1970s, Herbert Marcuse was considered one of the world's most important living theorists. Acclaimed throughout the world as a philosopher of liberation and revolution, Marcuse was a prominent figure in the Zeitgeist of the times, deeply influencing the New Left and oppositional movements. . . . Indeed, his books even reached a general public and he was discussed, attacked and celebrated in the mass media, as well as scholarly publications.

However, after his death in 1979 Marcuse's influence waned, in no small part because he was displaced by a new trend:

> Marcuse did not fit into the fashionable debates concerning modern and postmodern thought. Unlike Adorno, Marcuse did not anticipate the postmodern attacks on reason and enlightenment, and his dialectics were not "negative." Rather, Marcuse subscribed to the project of reconstructing reason and of positing utopian alternatives to the existing society—a dialectical imagination that has fallen out of favor in an era that rejects revolutionary thought and grand visions of liberation and social reconstruction. (Kellner, 1998, p. xiv)

People are often uncomfortable with critique of the society in which they live, expressing concern about specific problems such as corporate corruption or air pollution, but resisting identification of these problems as predictable outcomes of the structure and operation of society. This makes it more difficult to formulate broad, long-term solutions. Intellectual discomfort with patterns, structures, motivating forces, and outcomes has been intensified by the complexity of contemporary society, by postmodern questioning of foundational thought, and by globalized capitalist neoliberalism, with its media-driven, homogeneous popular culture. In this situation, the question is whether to accept the status quo or to challenge it by introducing critical imagination of societal alternatives into the discourse. This book suggests that the latter choice, for some people in specific circumstances, is preferable to passivity and acceptance.

As discussed in the first chapter, for several reasons critical theory has not had a significant impact within public administration. It is not the purpose of this book to bring the critical theory of the mid-twentieth century unchanged into the beginning of the twenty-first century, but to adapt useful conceptual elements from that body of work to contemporary circumstances. Marcuse's analysis of society, largely forgotten since the 1970s and criticized as simplistic and extreme, seems unnervingly prescient and pertinent today. When Marcuse's concerns are incorporated into the writing of contemporary theorists working with the complexities of today's society, they can become especially useful in conceptualizing alternative futures. It is my hope the exercise of critical imagination may appear to readers of this book to be the least we can do given the conditions that surround us.

Themes and Chapters

The material in this book was written over several years for presentation or publication. Each chapter addresses a particular question in the application of critical social theory to theory building and practice, with the later work emphasizing adaptation of Frankfurt thought to contemporary public administration. However, the sequence of chapters is not chronological, but reflects a flow of themes intended to draw the reader into a critical perspective on the context of public service. The reader will encounter some repetition in discussion of concepts, for example one-dimensionality, but each such discussion occurs in a different topical context and offers additional perspective.

Chapters 1, 2, and 3 introduce critical social theory and its application to research in public administration. Chapter 1 explores the history of use of critical theory in public administration, argues for its usefulness in the field, and presents the critical social theory framework of the book: contradiction, dialectic, and change; critical reason and imagination; and emancipation and self-determination. To illustrate differences between critical social theory and a currently well-known body of thought, it is contrasted with the postmodern pragmatism of Richard Rorty. Marcuse and Rorty share concerns about oppressive conditions in society, but their conclusions about what should be done are not at all alike.

Chapter 2 summarizes several features of Marcuse's work (democracy, the warfare state, the "research of total administration," and gender) along with his thoughts about features of a better society. The discussion of the research of total administration critiques positivist research that intends to describe the status quo and enable prediction and control, but instead applies an inappropriate "scientific" model from the natural sciences that is rarely useful for improving the practice of public service.

Scholarship that critically examines history, the ways we describe how the present was constructed, is the focus of Chapter 3. The narrative describes society as characterized by forms of oppression. Then, in a passage expressing a concern similar to John Kirlin's (1996) in a *Public Administration Review* article about "the big questions of public administration in a democracy," the narrative follows Curtis Ventriss in making the observation that:

> Given these assumptions about society, action, and history, the question becomes what academicians can or should do, within their scholarly work, in the service of meaningful change. We work in a field inclined toward the technical and instrumental, during a time when powerful forces breathe new life into the project of separating democratic will formation from administration, reanimating the politics-administration dichotomy that many thought had disappeared. These forces seek to collapse the two realms of thought in public administration, the social/political and the organizational/managerial, into one, the organizational/managerial. (Ventriss, 2000; in Box & King, 2000, p. 764)

The following four chapters address topics of importance to public administration practice, including discourse processes with citizens, the impact of administration on the public, and the problem of finding a "public" ready and willing to govern themselves if the opportunity is made available. In Chapter 4, a critical description of community politics is the context for examining the possibilities for public practitioners to facilitate citizen discourse in five local areas. "Discourse theory" in public administration has taken several forms. These are reviewed in Chapter 5, in which the potential for a pragmatic discourse model to create meaningful change is questioned on grounds that a critical perspective is needed to fully understand the political and economic setting of administration.

Without apology, Chapters 6 and 7 take a rather gloomy, critical turn. The argument in Chapter 6, that public practitioners should take care to avoid damage to "private lives," was written shortly before the events of September 2001 and seems even more pertinent today. One connection between concern for private lives and the framework of critical social theory is the description of the market-oriented societal context that shapes administrative action. To the extent those for whom the physical community is primarily a place for making profits are the influential people and elected officials who shape the actions of public agencies, there is potential for conflict with the interests of citizens who are primarily interested in the community as a place to live, as an environment of daily experience. Paradoxically, this concern about administrative impact on private lives parallels the classical liberal emphasis on "negative rights" (protection from action by the collectivity). However, the chapter does not intend, as do classical/neo liberals, to separate public and private matters so that "positive rights" (substantive equality and social justice) are off the public agenda.

Of key importance is the suggestion in Chapter 6 that public administrators should use imagination to conceptualize the lives of people in whose name they act. Private lives are grounded in material concerns about family and neighborhood, physical and social surroundings central to what Thomas Jefferson called "life, liberty and the pursuit of happiness." At the level of epistemology, this central concern for private lives presents a stark contrast between critical social theory and mainstream scholarly work. Critical social theory is not primarily about building knowledge upon statistically manipulated "data," it is about constructive change. The language of critical social theory may at times operate at a level of abstraction that obscures its purposes and grounding in daily experience. However, the reason for such theory is not abstract; it is practical, immediate, and solidly connected to the condition of the world. Certainly it is good if this effort benefits the academic enterprise, but this is not its primary purpose.

A central problem, however, addressed in Chapter 7, is that it is often difficult to find "a public" to assume responsibility for putting individual concerns on the public agenda. It is common in the literature of public administration to encounter the expectation that people want to participate in self-governance and that such involvement may make a difference in democratic processes and outcomes. Skepticism about the public's capacity to self-govern has been present throughout much of American history. In the current societal environment of advanced consumerist capitalism, it may be appropriate to acknowledge that this capacity has diminished to the point it is unrealistic to expect it to counter the forces arrayed against the idea of self-governance. The narrative of the chapter presents the example of design of local streetscapes as illustrative of the difficulty of overcoming the property-and-profit orientation that largely determines local public political and administrative life.

Chapter 7 also illustrates an important characteristic of the everyday application of a critical social theory framework. It can be applied to situations of class inequity and oppression that are the traditional concerns of "radical" thought, but limiting critical social theory to extreme examples of injustice, poverty, exploitation of labor, and so on, allows it to be conceptually excluded from settings more familiar to the middle-class majority. Central to the theme of the book is the idea that critical social theory can be useful in the most familiar and seemingly mundane circumstances of problem identification, decision making, and administrative implementation in the public sector.

The Critical Social Theory Framework

The contents of the book may seem relentlessly negative, but this is critical social theory, intended to identify contradictions between what is and what might be and to show the potential for constructive change. Though it might be comforting to find a blueprint for outcomes of application of the critical framework, there are only the preferences of people involved in specific acts of resistance against the status quo and efforts to create a better future. The focus here is on characterization of the societal context and application of a critical framework, a process of change. To the extent there are desired outcomes, they may be expressed in goals common to much of critical theory, which seeks to give people knowledge about their situation and alternatives and to offer them the means to create change, working toward a future that is peaceful and cooperative instead of aggressive and competitive. This implies changes in political and economic systems that will reduce coercion, injustice, inequality, and inequity.

The critical social theory framework of the book consists of three elements: contradiction, dialectic, and change; critical reason and imagination; and emancipation and self-determination. In practice, these three elements may or may not occur in consecutive order, as phases, depending on the point at which the thinking of involved citizens, practitioners, or academicians begins. The elements of the framework are discussed in detail later in the book, but it will be useful to briefly describe the concepts here.

Contradiction, dialectic, and change assume as a baseline the nature of society as described in the chapters of the book. In rough summary, this is a "one-dimensional" society, to use Marcuse's term, a society structured by the hegemonic global market (McSwite, 2002, p. 18). Liberal-capitalist democracy has become dominant to the point that knowledge of alternatives has faded; the sense that what-is-is-what-must-be affects not only thinking at the global or national level but also regions, communities, and neighborhoods, where economic efficiency and cost-benefit rationale push other public values to the margins of discourse and decision making, with consequent damage to individuals, societies, and the physical environment.

Control of government, in the past a seemingly complex matter of "who governs," a question to be debated by those favoring the view that an elite owns America and those who regard the public process as pluralist and inclusive, becomes more clearly a matter of naked economic interest. In such a setting, as McSwite (2002, p. 18) notes, "the market is in; government is out. The prevailing view is that as capitalism defeated the planned economies of socialism, so it also defeated the idea that government itself is essential." Though at times in the past this situation might have generated public unrest, today happy consumers accept goods and services in exchange for acquiescence.

This situation can, in specific times and places, generate awareness of contradiction between extant conditions and memories of what has been or values embedded in the cultural environment. Terry Cooper (1998, p. 176) provides a sample of such values in the American context: "the beneficial effect of a pluralism of interests, the creative possibilities in conflict, the sovereignty of the public, the rights of the minority, the importance of citizen participation in government, the societal values of freedom of expression, and the centrality of justice in the relationship between the people and their government." Any current conditions contain within them the possibility of change, from today's seemingly permanent social structures and practices to potential alternative futures. This potential dialectical change can be facilitated with critical reason and imagination, giving people the knowledge they need to be emancipated from one-dimensional thought, allowing them to envision alternatives that move them closer to the ideal of self-determining their collective future. This may sound much like a typical strategic planning process, but it is qualitatively different. Rather than searching for competitive advantage within existing societal systems, the critical framework suggests questioning those systems and working for basic change.

The presentation here of a critical framework is not about specific techniques, such as creating workable discourse settings or countering the influence of private interests. These things are important, but the current exercise is about applying a critical social framework to assist with scholarship and practice. Desired outcomes, certainly in the short term, need not involve totalizing or immediate change in broad economic, political, and governmental practices. Dialectical change is likely never ending. Earlier critical thought envisioned sudden revolutionary change from the inequality, injustice, competitiveness, and violence of capitalist society to a society that would be cooperative, egalitarian, nonviolent, and oriented toward free and creative individual development.

Today, the likelihood of significant large-scale social change seems more remote than ever. This does not mean the goal of constructive change is invalid, but that actions, processes, and expectations will be mostly local and small-scale, and that participants will tend to experience change as a process rather than a destination. Change based on critical social theory may be contrasted with isolated reformist responses to especially unpleasant situations, without plan or long-range purpose. This is the occasional, random reduction of injustice advocated by the progressive left (Rorty, 1998b), intended to shave the rough edges off capitalist society without challenging its fundamental premises. A critical approach, in contrast, involves a systematic analysis of societal conditions and a framework for action guided by normative purpose. It is probably never ending, in part because the task of changing one-dimensional society is incredibly large, but also because any condition to which it might be changed would also be subject to dialectical change. Given this characteristic of dialectical change and because it seems pointless today to claim knowledge of absolutes, we understand there is no perfect, foundational, utopian ideal, and we need not be afflicted with "naive expectations about the autonomy of reason from political reality or the capacity of reason to defeat naked power" (Cohen & Rogers, 2003, p. 253).

Herbert Marcuse described, in a way few others have, the nature and effects of late-modern society. Though he held to the dream of radical, large-scale change, he recognized the potential of local, small-scale action. It would be interesting to know how he would respond to conditions in the early twenty-first century. It is difficult to believe he would entirely abandon hope for fundamental change in society, change resulting in different perspectives on human fulfillment, work, and the relationship of people to the physical environment. However, he might be pushed by circumstances to acknowledge we live in a "postsocialist" world in which the best a radical reformer might expect, at least in the short term, is movement toward an "egalitarian-democratic" society (Cohen & Rogers, 2003, p. 253). This would not be an insignificant achievement, nor is it without precedent in historical thought. It shares much with the purposes of the Leveller and Digger movements during the English Civil War of the 1640s, and also with the "republican" thought of many Americans during the founding era of the late eighteenth century (Box, 2004, pp. 29–33). Critical social theory encourages academicians and practitioners to view social structures and practices as vehicles of domination, repression, and manipulation, but also as potential starting points for meaningful social change.

— 1 —

Critical Imagination in a Postmodern Environment

Critical theory has been marginal in public administration, though it offers critique of public institutions and possibilities for a better future. Among several reasons for this, it may be that its normative vision of social change challenges the status quo and threatens the economic and political equilibrium. The sections below summarize characteristics of critical social theory, note ways it has been used in public administration, and contrast it with postmodern pragmatism to illustrate the difference between critical social theory and well-known contemporary thought. Critical theory may be even more valuable today than in the past, as one-dimensional society and postmodernism close off description of societal conditions and use of imagination to create a better future.

Public administration is a field of knowledge with uncertain boundaries. Public administration scholars are hesitant to call it a discipline, and, for lack of theories indigenous to the field, they borrow many of their conceptual frameworks from other areas of knowledge (for example, from business administration, theories of management, leadership, employee motivation, and so on; and from political science and economics, theories about structural arrangements such as representation, accountability, and legitimacy). In such a field, one would think a body of theory that offers critique of public institutions plus a vision of a better future would appeal to writers. Critical theory does these things, but it appears infrequently in the literature of public administration.

Several possible reasons might be suggested for the apparent failure of critical theory to have a significant impact in public administration: the theories most commonly used in public administration operate at the micro-level of organizational management rather than as broad social theory; critical theory tends to surface in public administration during times of social turmoil and change then falls into obscurity during times of relative stability; an instrumental field of practice does not need abstract thought; and, the times are now postmodern, rendering theories based on Enlightenment humanism obsolete.

These are potentially viable reasons for the scarcity of critical theory in public administration, but they seem unsatisfying, incomplete. There have been opportunities for critical theory to take hold in public administration, as discussed below, but it nevertheless appears only in the work of a few. Critical thought has failed to influence public administration theory because its normative vision of social change challenges the status quo and threatens the economic and political equilibrium. Public administration theory and practice operate within the context of intensifying global capitalism, and the logic of the market permeates private and public life, pushing back bodies of thought that suggest alternative ways of organizing social and governmental relationships. As this circumstance becomes dominant, critique and discussion of alternative ways to organize relationships between individuals and institutions fades in perceived importance and relevance, though it may actually be more pertinent than ever.

The sections below summarize characteristics of critical social theory, note ways it has been used in public administration, and contrast critical theory with postmodern pragmatism to illustrate the difference between critical social theory and well-known contemporary thought. The theme is that critical theory can be a useful way to conceptualize the place of public administration in society for theorists and practitioners concerned about social conditions and the possibilities for meaningful change. This is not an argument that seeks to put critical social theory in a position of primacy by devaluing other approaches to public administration—at most, this body of theory will likely appeal to a niche audience in public administration. The point is to offer it to that audience in hopes that it may foster constructive change.

Critical Social Theory

The term *critical theory* can be used in a broad, inclusive way, masking significant differences in approach. A number of writers offer critique of society and some include in their writing elements of what has come to be thought of as critical theory. People only tangentially familiar with critical theory may think of it as an antiquated body of thought based on a crude, discredited Marxism. For our purposes here, critical theory is associated with the Frankfurt school beginning in the 1920s and extending through the later work of principal members Max Horkheimer, Theodor Adorno, and Herbert Marcuse, in the 1960s and 1970s (see Jay, 1973). The term *critical theory* is also applied to writers whose work began in the early part of the twentieth century, such as Georg Lukacs and Antonio Gramsci, as well as to later twentieth-century writers such as Jürgen Habermas.

Because of differences in approach between authors and changes in the work of individual authors over time, it is difficult to construct a unitary narrative of critical theory. It will be helpful to identify a few common characteristics in this body of work, recognizing that not all authors treat them the same, or even agree on their status within critical theory. At its broadest, critical theory is grounded in the Enlightenment, eighteenth-century thought in Europe and America that used science, reason, and individual self-determination to cast off religious and governmental authority. History came to be seen as linear, progressive, and leading to human improvement as people would conquer nature and overcome the limitations of resource scarcity. The nineteenth-century writing of Karl Marx was a reaction against the effects of capitalism, the social and economic form society had taken since the Enlightenment, and critical theory can be described as a "category of sociological thought" that developed from the work of Marx (Burrell & Morgan, 1979, p. 283). Though critical theory has in important ways moved beyond Marx as times have changed and problems have been identified in his work, it includes the three characteristics discussed below.

Contradiction, Dialectic, and Change

A primary characteristic of critical theory is the idea that social systems change over time because of built-in tensions, or contradictions, between how they are and how they could be. Examples include the contrasting preferences of capitalists and workers, bureaucrats and citizens, land developers and people concerned about the living environment, people pleased with the current distribution of income and wealth in society and those who would change it, and so on. Each such systemic contradiction is "inherent in and cannot be solved without modifying, or 'moving beyond,' the basic structure in which it occurs" (Mills, 1962, p. 83). The current "basic structure," or status quo, is the surface reality "given" to us by sense perception. It is this surface reality that is most frequently studied by scientists and scholars and accepted as "the way it is."

Horkheimer called the exercise of documenting the given "traditional theory" (1972, pp. 188–243). Beyond the static knowledge of traditional theory and inherent in the characteristics of all things is the potential for transformation of the given into something different. Critical theory explores this potential, as it "shows the relationships between ideas and theoretical positions and their social environment, and thus attempts to contextualize, or historicize, ideas in terms of their roots in social processes" (Kellner, 1989, p. 45). Because it studies ways the given may be changed to the benefit of humankind, critical theory "is oppositional and involved in a struggle for social change and the unification of theory and practice" (p. 46).

The process of acquiring knowledge of alternatives to the status quo and encouraging constructive change is dialectical. The Frankfurt school's use of the Hegelian concept of dialectic is not conceptually foundational and does not involve a predetermined outcome. In agreement with writers such as Lukacs, Korsch, and Gramsci, Frankfurt theorists rejected "objectivistic Marxism," a type of Marxist thought that emphasized "economic laws and objective social conditions" (Kellner, 1989, p. 11). Their version of dialectic "stressed instead complex, contradictory sets of social relations and struggles in a specific historical era, whose trajectory could not be determined with certainty in advance" (p. 11). According to Douglas Kellner, Marcuse's use of the dialectical method regarded its object of study as part of a historical process; it is a method that perceives, quoting Marcuse, "every developing form in the river of movement. . . . It considers its object as being in a state of becoming and passing away, as necessarily arising from a determinate historical situation, related to human existence rooted in this situation" (in Kellner, 1984, p. 52).

Critical Reason and Imagination

One might think "reason" to be a good thing; in everyday speech it is complimentary to say one is reasonable and uncomplimentary to say one is unreasonable. However, reason has become a negative idea in much scholarly writing, a symbol of the way the Enlightenment project of creating a better world with rational thought has been twisted into means-end instrumental reason, used to maintain social conditions that benefit a few at the expense of others.

Martin Jay notes that Frankfurt theorists stressed reason and gave the term a specific meaning derived from Kant and Hegel. This meaning contrasts reason with "understanding," which is the common-sense perception of the world. "To the understanding, the world consisted of finite entities identical only with themselves and totally opposed to all other things. It thus failed to penetrate immediacy to grasp the dialectical relations beneath the surface." In contrast, reason "signified a faculty that went beyond mere appearances," exploring "a deeper reality" (Jay, 1973, p. 60), knowledge of the contradictory opposite(s) of things, people, and situations, into which they may change over time.

The problem was that modern reason was Enlightenment gone bad—reason that had served the goal of freedom had become a force for protecting the damaging features of advanced capitalism. Horkheimer and Adorno wrote in 1944 in *Dialectic of Enlightenment* they remained "convinced . . . that social freedom is inseparable from enlightened thought" (p. xiii). People must be free to reason for themselves and reasoning for themselves is the path to freedom. But, reason and enlightenment had become instruments of oppression. Horkheimer concluded *Eclipse of Reason* in 1947 by writing, "If by enlightenment and intellectual progress we mean the freeing of man from superstitious belief in evil forces, in demons and fairies, in blind fate—in short, the emancipation from fear—then denunciation of what is currently called reason is the greatest service reason can render" (1947, p. 187).

Despite this depressing view of the contemporary use of reason as a vehicle of constructive social change, Marcuse wished to rescue reason and with it the possibility that people could consciously choose the future. Part of this attempt involved an attack on common sense and positivism as examples of instrumental reason that preserves the given reality, obscuring the potential for change. Common sense and positivism contain and neutralize critique as they induce "thought to be satisfied with the facts, to renounce any transgression beyond them, and to bow to the given state of affairs" (Marcuse, 1941, p. 27). However, "if the task of theoretical analysis is more and other than a descriptive one—if the task is to *comprehend,* to *recognize* the facts for what they are, what they 'mean' for those who have been given them as facts and who have to live with them. . . ." then, "recognition of facts is critique of facts" (Marcuse, 1964, p. 118).

The central issue is whether current structures, institutions, and practices in society should be perceived as given, fixed, value free, virtually inevitable, or whether they should be considered malleable material to work with in reshaping reality. From the Enlightenment concept of conceptualizing change, reason has become instead a narrative told by those who want things to stay as they are. As Ben Agger (1992, p. 139) writes, "Marcuse suggests that what is an apparently value-free rationality of purposiveness, pragmatism, technique, and efficiency actually contains the substantive ethos of profit maximization and domination."

Though critical theorists believe that reason has been used in support of systems of domination and control, some also think people can use reason to imagine a different future. The status of reason, especially in what may be considered a condition of "postmodernity," remains an open question, but critical theorists who understand the "dialectic of enlightenment" and are committed to a nonfoundational, historically based process of change may seek to reconstruct *critical reason* as a counter to contemporary instrumental rationality. As Marcuse (1968, p. 225) put it, "technical reason is the social reason ruling a given society and can be changed in its very structure." Critical reason in practice involves the dialectical use of imagination and fantasy to envision a better future (pp. 154–155).

Emancipation and Self-determination

Today, philosophical postmodernism questions the existence of "the subject," the self-aware, self-reflective, thinking, feeling individual, substituting instead a person who is a product of larger patterns and forces in society, a fragmented individual "with a disparate personality and a potentially confused identity" (Rosenau, 1992, p. 55). The fading of the subject is not a new thought, but may be traced back at least to the nineteenth-century writing of Nietzsche. A weakened subject can be found in the work of Jürgen Habermas, who turned from the Frankfurt school's emphasis on consciousness to the characteristics of communication in discourse settings (Rasmussen, 1990, pp. 24–26), and it can be found within the original Frankfurt group. According to Agger (1992, p. 233), Adorno suggested the subject had been largely obliterated by the dominant ideology of society, becoming "nearly impotent, voiceless. . . , a trivial and forgotten moment." Marcuse hoped the subject could be reinvigorated, but given the nature of contemporary industrial society he was pessimistic. The same corporations that dictate the characteristics of the workplace shape the individual's leisure time, which becomes a reflection of "the qualities, attitudes, values, behavior belonging to his station in his society," so that "his leisure activity or passivity will simply be a prolongation or recreation of his social performance" (2001b, p. 74). This "ingression" of market society "into all spheres of the individual existence" makes it difficult to imagine individuals as freely choosing, autonomous subjects.

The view within critical theory that humans are "socially constructed" can be found in Marx's writing from the mid-nineteenth century: "the human being is in the most literal sense a political animal, not merely a gregarious animal, but an animal which can individuate itself only in the midst of society" (in Tucker, 1972, p. 223). The social construction perspective is reflected in the work of Frankfurt theorists, for example Marcuse (1968, pp. 77–79). Frankfurt critical theory recognizes the concrete temporal and cultural specificity of the individual consciousness—values and perceptions are shaped by the time and society in which we live—but ultimately the measure of society is, as it has been since the Enlightenment, its effect on people, on their happiness and sense of freedom to determine the future.

Critical theorists tend to be wary of describing utopian visions of a society freed from economic domination and inequalities of power, wealth, and class. They recognize that the Marxian moment of a possible uprising of the workers to create a new society has long passed. One view of what has taken its place (a view considered extreme by some; see Kellner, 1989, p. 203) is Marcuse's (1964) "one-dimensional" society, a capitalist system based on destruction of natural resources in pursuit of profit, supported by hostility toward supposed enemies who would threaten the consumer culture and its benefits for the controlling class (pp. 48–55). This system is reinforced by corporate-delivered entertainment providing the distraction of meaningless "sport, fun, and fad" (Marcuse, 2001b, p. 74), while the nation finds, and if necessary, kills, those who endanger the comfortable system (Marcuse, 2001c, p. 157).

Faced with these circumstances, it would be understandable for critical theorists to abandon the idea of radical change in societal institutions and practices that would allow for greater human freedom and self-determination. Jürgen Habermas, a student of the first-generation Frankfurt theorists, has given up social analysis based on economic contradiction, critique of ideology, and utopian vision (Braaten, 1991, p. 154). The earlier Frankfurt theorists became pessimistic about the possibilities for meaningful change, but retained hope for "something that might be attained, an object to be strived for" (Alway, 1995, p. 127). Marcuse never completely lost hope in the future, which for him would be a nonrepressive civilization that would include use of technology that reduces the time devoted to work required for obtaining the necessities of life, thus freeing human creative capacities (Kellner, 1984, pp. 176–178). Society would be peaceful rather than aggressive, careful with use of nature and resources, and governance would take place in a setting of decentralization and decision making by the people, a "libertarian socialism" (Kellner, 1984, p. 322). Interestingly, this latter concept finds parallels in contemporary democratic and discourse theory.

Critical Theory in Public Administration

It may be argued that "administrative neutrality" is the foundational myth of public administration. Although public professionals often significantly influence public policy making and policy implementation, there remains a societal expectation that public administrators receive already-created policy direction and implement it while exercising relatively little discretion. In keeping with the preferences of some economic and political elites, "new public management" reinforces this myth by narrowing the scope of public practice to cost-efficient implementation; simultaneously, positivist research methodologies encourage a static view of the public sphere.

A continuum may be described of public administrator involvement in shaping the creation and implementation of public policy. At one end is uninvolvement, the "ideal" of administrative neutrality. At the other end is the administrator as fully involved policy actor seeking to influence the knowledge, opinions, and decisions of citizens, elected officials, and peers. Critical theory provides an opening for conceptualization and practice that acknowledges the value-based, normative character of public administration. The public professional who perceives contradiction between current public practices and a future with reduced inequity and oppression may use critical theory as a guide for taking action to create social change.

Traditional "classical liberals" (today, "neoliberals") object to involvement by public professionals in the policy process. Nostalgically, they envision a very small government from an imagined earlier era when pluralist politics could be relied upon to protect the individual from abuse by the rich and powerful. If this era ever existed, it has long since disappeared. Like the communitarian's imagined past of solidarity and community, the pioneer society of rugged individuals protected by a set of "negative rights" has given way to large-scale urban, industrial, technological interrelatedness with almost unimaginable inequalities of wealth and power. Now, to assume that neutrality is possible is to fail to understand that neutrality itself is a value-laden choice. To fail to consciously choose a role in social change is to relinquish initiative to those with the energy and sense of purpose to maintain or shape society as they think it should be.

Public administration writing is often focused on specific areas of practice such as budgeting, facilitating citizen involvement in decision making, and so on. It often does not make explicit the historical/political/economic context that frames and constrains action. However, as John Kirlin (1996) has argued, the "big questions" of the societal environment of public administration are a crucial part of theory and practice. Critical theory suggests it is useful to understand the societal surroundings in relation to, at least, the three elements noted in the sections above. What is the observed contradiction between existing circumstances and the potential alternatives, especially as considered from the perspective of historical values of the society and its culture? Within a dialectical process of change, movement from what is to what could be, what choices are most appropriate to serve valued ends such as emancipation and self-determination?

Within the category of public administration literature that goes beyond describing the status quo, much of what is found advocates moderate, incremental reform rather than dramatic changes in institutions or practices. There is an implicit assumption that the current legal, political, and economic framework is acceptable in broad terms, that perceived needs for change are limited to incremental adjustments that, so to speak, "shave the rough edges" off liberal-capitalist society, meliorating abuses that many if not most people would agree are too extreme. A good example is the shift in governmental posture toward labor-management relations in the first half of the twentieth century, from protecting the profits of capitalists by using armed officers to attack protesting laborers, to allowing workers to organize for collective bargaining.

Reformist writing in public administration often urges change that encourages emancipation and self-determination, though it operates within the given system. The "new public administration" of the 1960s and 1970s (not to be confused with new public management) suggested that public professionals encourage greater "social equity," a goal requiring some redistribution of wealth and power in society. H. George Frederickson's (1980, p. 37) narrative describing the conceptual basis of new public administration recognized that government is controlled by the powerful and discriminates against those who lack power and money to resist. Public administrators should seek to alleviate these conditions to some extent because they create "anger and militancy" and may lead to calls for public employees "to oppress the deprived" (p. 38). The theoretical backdrop of this view is John Rawls's "theory of justice," a meliorist ethical approach based on "welfare state liberalism" (A. Ryan, 1997, p. 296). Pushed only a bit further, new public administration could be framed within an analysis of contradiction between existing political/economic systems and systems largely devoid of the abuses found within the liberal welfare state. This, however, would be a thoroughly radical thought in the current environment of institutions and practices. Even in the atmosphere of transformation in the 1960s and 1970s, the new public administration premise that public employees could promote change within the political/economic order was "far out" in relation to mainstream practice.

The communication theory of Habermas is the most commonly used version of critical theory in public administration today. Habermas writes that public discourse is distorted by unequal power relationships introduced into discourse by the nature of the surrounding liberal-capitalist welfare state. Examples of distorted communication can be found in areas such as mass media and issues of social welfare (Braaten, 1991, pp. 141–156). Habermas believes that consensual, distortion-free communication would be a progressive step toward reviving Enlightenment rationality in defense of democracy (Best & Kellner, 1991, pp. 240–241). These ideas have been influential, but questions have arisen about the efficacy of distortion-free communication as a way to change society as a whole. Also, as Chantal Mouffe (2000, p. 104) argues, democracy is not a search for distortion-free consensus, but is instead a matter of contestation and dispute, "a vibrant clash of democratic political positions" that is ongoing, dynamic, unresolvable. In later work Habermas has moved away from critical theory toward reformist liberalism (Alway, 1995, p. 126), but the idea of undistorted communication as a critical tool for social change has been important in public administration.

Robert Denhardt (1981a) suggested that a critical approach to organizational theory would be useful in public administration. Denhardt reviewed the origins of critical theory, from Hegel and Marx to the Frankfurt theorists, but focused on Habermas. He emphasized the Habermasian concern about supposedly value-free science and efficiency and urged attention to the "larger historical and normative context" (p. 633) of public organizations as part of a critical examination of bureaucracy and its relationships with clients. In an article in the *Journal of the American Planning Association,* John Forester (1980, p. 278) applied Habermasian concepts to planning practice, identifying four "norms of pragmatic communication" which are "usually taken for granted": to speak comprehensively; to speak sincerely; to speak legitimately, in context; and to speak the truth. When planners violate these norms with distorted communication, the result can be community residents who exhibit "puzzlement, mistrust, anger, and disbelief" (p. 278).

Turning from Habermas to critical theory more broadly, Jay White and Guy Adams argued for greater attention to critical research approaches in the preface to their 1994 book on research in public administration. Relatively few people have done so, though examples may be noted. Denhardt's book *In the Shadow of Organization* (1981b) used a critical approach to imagine organizations better suited to the creative, human needs of employees. Guy Adams, Priscilla Bowerman, Kenneth Dolbeare, and Camilla

Stivers (1990, p. 227) criticized the emphasis in American democracy on procedural justice and the corresponding inattention to substantive matters of economic justice. They hoped to "restore and develop the socially revealing, integrated political-economic perspective; to recapture the full version of democracy that is consistent with such a view of the social world; and to seek its realization in practice." Richard Box (1995) used critical concepts from Marcuse, Habermas, Harvey Molotch's (1976; Logan & Molotch, 1987) neo-Marxist "growth machine" theory of urban politics, and case examples to construct a discourse-facilitative model of public professional practice; this theme was developed further in the book *Citizen Governance* (Box, 1998). Lisa Zanetti and Adrian Carr (1997, p. 208) wrote that critical theory "provides an ethical impulse toward substantive equality and democracy." They believed that "critical theory has much to offer the field of public administration" and its intent "is to create self-reflective consciousness such that theory and practice become one." Drawing from several critical theorists and in particular Antonio Gramsci and his notion of "organic intellectuals," Zanetti (1997) offered a model of public administration researchers and practitioners as transformative change agents.

Several articles and books in public administration and related fields have used concepts with critical elements though they are not explicitly built upon critical theory. Richard Box and Cheryl Simrell King (2000) identified such works in the historical study of public affairs, for example Camilla Stivers' *Bureau Men and Settlement Women: Constructing Public Administration in the Progressive Era* (2000a) and Gordon Wood's *The Creation of the American Republic 1776–1787* (1969).

The Need for Critical Theory Today

Since critical theory has occupied only a small niche in public administration, it is appropriate to question why it now deserves additional attention. This could be difficult to answer in a time of prosperous, globalized liberal-capitalist society. Because critical theory threatens the status quo by focusing on discordant, troubling aspects of society and how they might be changed, people may find it unattractive and not especially useful. Two aspects of the contemporary condition, postmodernism and one-dimensionality, may contribute to this perception of critical theory.

Postmodernism provides a corrective to modernist thought that ignores differences, marginalizing certain people and practices as "other" (Agger, 2002, p. 212). In public administration, it draws attention to the lack of foundational concepts to ground theory, encouraging theorists to confront the assumptions inherent in their work (Fox & Miller, 1995). Useful features of postmodern thought such as antifoundationalism can also make it difficult to formulate coherent theories. Postmodernism resists large-scale, holistic social thought (metanarratives), complicating description of the societal backdrop to administrative practice. Postmodern skepticism about foundationalism and metanarrative makes critical theory unappealing, especially for those who think of it in caricature, as crude Marxism from the early twentieth century. The issue becomes whether critical theory remains viable in a late modern or postmodern world and whether it can be adapted to the present.

Descriptions of contemporary society rendered by critical theorists have changed over several decades as circumstances have changed, though the central concern continues to be the impact of the capitalist economic system on human life and the physical environment. The Frankfurt theorists wrote from their observations of fascism, authoritarian communism, and capitalism beginning in the period between World Wars I and II. As hope for revolutionary change in dominant systems faded in mid-century, critical descriptions of economics, politics, and culture reflected a sense of resignation in the face of powerful and pervasive conditions that overwhelmed the minority whose progressive ideals were out of step with the times.

In the 1960s and 1970s, Marcuse worked to keep alive a sense of the potential for change despite what he called the *one-dimensional* nature of society. This concept is exactly the sort of totalizing metanarrative postmodernism rejects; it describes a society so completely structured around advanced consumerist capitalism that virtually no one is aware of or can envision alternatives. One-dimensionality may seem paradoxical or self-contradictory, since we, or at least the "we" who live in advanced Western democracies, think there is complete freedom to contemplate alternatives and advocate for change. However, a critical examination of contemporary conditions might suggest that Marcuse is correct, the economic and political system has repressed both knowledge of alternatives and the impulse to think in dialectical form of possible change.

Steven Best and Douglas Kellner (2001, p. 1) offer an interesting description of the times in *The Postmodern Adventure*. They characterize recent decades as a "great transformation," an "upheaval in an era marked by technological revolution and the global restructuring of capitalism." This "globalization has produced a world economic system and trade laws that protect transnational corporations at the expense of human life, biodiversity, and the environment," and its effects include "heightened exploitation of labor, corporate downsizing, and greater levels of unemployment, inequality, and insecurity." David Harvey (2000, p. 220) describes the environmental consequences of the global economic system as quantitative shifts in "scientific knowledge and engineering capacities, industrial output, waste generation, invention of new chemical compounds, urbanization, population growth, international trade, fossil fuel consumption, resource extraction, habitat modification," resulting in "massive environmental changes . . . some distinctly harmful to us and others unnecessarily harmful to other species."

This is not a postmodern condition different from advanced capitalism, it *is* the mature, pervasive, globalized form of advanced capitalism. The resulting psychological effect is that "the world we experience appears to us to exhaust all possible worlds" (Agger, 2002, p. 3). This sounds like a fully realized form of Marcuse's one-dimensionality.

The situation today presents an odd contrast with the times that generated critical social theory in past decades. The world is peaceful in comparison to the upheaval of world war, but there is instability and violence in many places. People in "developed" nations with stable institutions lead safe and prosperous lives, reflected in their public sector theory and practice. They have the luxury of concentrating on cost-efficiency of service delivery in public organizations in the (presumed) absence of pressing substantive matters from earlier times, such as poverty, racism, and environmental degradation. It is important to consider whether the developed Western democracies have in fact achieved such an advanced state of being, and equally important to ask about conditions in the rest of the world while the rich nations enjoy their wealth.

Pragmatism and Phantasy

For the Frankfurt theorists, much contemporary scholarly research is questionable because of its positivist fixation on the extant, the given, the compilation of alleged "facts" documenting the socioeconomic status quo. Though early scientific method served as a means to critique superstition and dogma (Kellner, 1984, p. 139), it developed later into "positivism, the philosophy of common sense," which rejected thinking beyond existing facts (Marcuse, 1941, p. 113). Frankfurt critical theorists used the philosophy of American pragmatism as an example of thinking that fails to go beyond instrumental implementation of the status quo. According to Horkheimer (1947, pp. 41–57), pragmatism rejects theory as guide to practice, so that no goal is inherently better than another except to the extent it can be proved by experiment to be useful. This "reduction of reason to a mere instrument" (p. 54) results in "a doctrine that holds not that our expectations are fulfilled and our actions successful because our ideas are true, but rather that our ideas are true because our expectations are fulfilled and our actions successful" (p. 42).

Critical theory, in contrast, projects beyond the present, because "in the theoretical reconstruction of the social process, the critique of current conditions and the analysis of their tendencies necessarily include future-oriented components" (Marcuse, 1968, p. 145). In so doing, it engages the imagination, the use of "phantasy" (Marcuse's spelling). However, "owing to its unique capacity to 'intuit' an object though the latter be not present and to create something new out of given material of cognition, imagination denotes a considerable degree of independence from the given, of freedom amid a world of unfreedom" (p. 154). This does not mean unlimited, foundational, idealistic, or pointless thought, but thought that searches for alternatives to the present within the historical possibilities available to people in specific, material circumstances. To search for "a more beautiful and happier world" requires, as Marcuse wrote, "independence from the given"; thus, it will not appeal to everyone and may be looked upon as "the prerogative of children and fools" (p. 154).

A more recent threat to critical theory and practice, postmodernism, makes it difficult to identify societal trends, resist dominance, and envision a better future. Postmodern thought may find inequity, oppressive power, and the false appearances of hyperreal media and culture to be inevitable characteristics of society, while critical theory would describe them as the results of actions taken by those with money and power. If people regard such things as beyond their control, they are likely to regress into a passivity resembling the human condition the Enlightenment arose to reverse, a condition of superstitious fatalism in the face of poorly understood forces. Such passivity is in contrast to dialectical thought, critical reason, and emancipation/self-determination; though critical theorists recognize the magnitude of the challenge of social change in contemporary conditions, they choose not to "fall prey to a nihilistic skepticism" (Kellner, 1989, p. 231).

In the scholarly study of public administration, a concern may be raised that academicians are settling into acceptance of one-dimensionality in research, a kind of "conceptual cleansing" in which critical thought about the role of the public sector in the broader society is vanishing. Though Frankfurt theorists used pragmatism to critique common-sense, positivist thinking, Frankfurt critical theory and contemporary postmodern pragmatism share a concern for human freedom from the cruelty and oppression that often results from inequalities of wealth and power. Pragmatist Richard

Rorty's work may be used to illustrate the similarities and differences in Frankfurt and so-called postmodern theorizing, highlighting a concern that today's theory has difficulty moving beyond the given.

Rorty's approaches to philosophy, politics, and social analysis are intensely controversial. He has been dismissed and ridiculed for his alleged simplifications, errors of fact, and irrationalist positions; despite, or perhaps because of this, he is one of the best-known American intellectuals of the day. Though Rorty (2001, p. 22) does not like the term "postmodern," calling it "exasperating," and noting that it can be used to "refer to an attitude of political hopelessness" (p. 20), his attack on philosophical foundationalism has made him an icon of postmodern thought.

Contemporary critical theorist Ben Agger (2002, p. 213) would like to deal with what he calls "the failure of the Enlightenment" by rebuilding "the goal of modernity," which is "social, political, and economic institutions that serve human needs." Critical theorist Douglas Kellner (1989, pp. 225–233) believes that socialism and democracy are compatible and that corrective action in liberal-capitalist society can be taken in areas such as consumer protection, education, and peace. Rorty, though, has no use for critique of the capitalist socioeconomic system. For him, capitalism is not the problem, so that, "unless some new metanarrative eventually replaces the Marxist one, we shall have to characterize the source of human misery in such untheoretical and banal ways as 'greed,' 'selfishness,' and 'hatred'" (Rorty, 1998a, p. 235).

This use of words is interesting. Marcuse described the capitalist economic system as creating "misery, cruelty, and repression" (Marcuse & Popper, 1976, p. 101)—not identical, but close in meaning. To avoid following the trail of evidence to the source of such conditions, Rorty relies on observed, but unexplained, human behavior. It is observed because it permeates human practices, but unexplained because a postmodernist cannot attribute such behavior to a causal factor such as cultural conditioning or human nature, much less the economic-political system.

Rather than link Enlightenment philosophy to Enlightenment political ends, Rorty would split them apart, so that the philosophical project of "finding a new, comprehensive, world-view which would replace God with Nature and Reason" would be scrapped, while the political project of creating what Rorty calls "a heaven on earth; a world without caste, class, or cruelty" (2001, p. 19), would be retained, not because it is "true" in a universal sense, but because people from a certain historical-political culture find this project worthwhile. Rorty (1999, p. 232) acknowledges that "the Marxists were right about at least one thing: the central political questions are those about the relations between rich and poor." He writes that human nature is a social construction rather than given by nature (Rorty, 1989, pp. 184–185; 2000, pp. 61–62), but nevertheless "the people who have already got their hands on money and power will lie, cheat and steal in order to make sure that they and their descendants monopolize both for ever" (Rorty, 1999, p. 206). How "natural" must something be to continue "for ever"? If such behavior is shaped by society and is not hard-wired in the human brain by evolution, what sort of societal change must take place to produce more desirable behavior?

Despite differences between critical theorists and the leftist-postmodern Rorty, their concerns about society are strikingly similar. Rorty's vision of an egalitarian utopia without class or caste in which people are free to create themselves as they please shares characteristics of Marcuse's libertarian socialism in which "reality no longer need be defined by the debilitating competition for social survival and advancement" (Marcuse, 1969, p. 5). Rorty emphasizes his lack of foundational intent as a distinction between his ideas and those of a generalized group he labels "Marxists." However, the Frankfurt theorists locate normative purpose in the concrete historical experience of particular peoples and cultures, not in timeless assumptions (Horkheimer, 1972)—Rorty's observation is an overgeneralization.

Rorty takes the position that public matters do not require theory. He thinks philosophy spoils public debate, which should consist of what he calls "as plain, blunt, public, easy-to-handle language as possible" (Rorty, 1996, p. 45). However, stripping ideas out of public discourse is a way of keeping the public space safely one-dimensional, denying that people are capable of conceptualizing their situation beyond incremental reform. What's left in Rorty's public sphere is a collection of people, for example Americans, who share common commitments and values and make collective decisions based on what they feel at the moment is good to do. Unfortunately, this nonreflective decision making, limited to what Rorty (1999, p. 198) describes as "the interest of a historically conditioned community," can, as Stephen Kautz (1996, p. 174) put it, "easily slide into the ugly and thuggish self-satisfaction of those who suppose they already know what they need to know." Rorty does not want this to happen; in his utopia, "nobody will be humiliated by bullies—neither by slaveowners, nor by factory owners, nor by husbands. The elimination of vast social and economic inequalities will help people treat one another decently. Mankind will finally escape from the thuggery of the schoolyard, put away childish things, and be morally mature" (Rorty, 2001, p. 23). But because he wants to avoid thinking about significant change in institutions and practices, this vision will likely remain private and ineffectual.

This brief comparison of critical theory and postmodern pragmatism is not intended to refute or reject Rorty's work as a whole. His ideas are used here as a foil for critical theory to illustrate that describing conditions in society is different from thinking about social change, and that lack of connection between them can lead to inaction. Limiting scholarly work to documenting the given and avoiding reflection on contradiction, alternative futures, and intended change, strengthens the one-dimensionality of scholarship. That may be especially problematic in public administration, a field that focuses attention on issues that can be addressed only through modification of institutions and practices.

Conclusion: A Critical Revival?

A turn in scholarly thought away from social theory and the project of human freedom may reflect the materially comfortable situation of some people in advanced nations. Worldwide, the daily lives of most people are focused on making a living and evading domination in the public sphere, the workplace, or in private life based on class, gender, race, ethnic identity, or the whims of dictators, criminals, abusive bosses, or intrusive government officials. It remains a material world. The conditions of life for many consist of basic matters of negotiating one's way through constraints based in no small part on the unequal distribution of material resources and the systems of power that support it. To claim that power and domination simply *are,* like the wind and the waves, or that institutional structures, broad patterns of social practice, and matters of economics and geographic place are not valid objects of concern, can be regarded as expressing the perspective of the privileged and protected strata of the developed countries. This is a narrow, ahistorical perspective that ignores recent human history as well as current conditions, in communities, in nations, and globally.

Given societal conditions and the nature of research and practice in public administration, the conceptual framework of critical social theory (contradiction, dialectic, and change; critical reason and imagination; emancipation and self-determination) offers promise for those scholars who wish to critique the status quo of professional practice in public organizations, with intent to imagine better options for the future. Much scholarly literature is devoted to studying behavior in public organizations and suggesting ways it may be controlled. This is useful, but it does not offer public administration practitioners or theorists ideas for crafting constructive roles in society. Because public employees are influential in the processes of creating and implementing public policy, it seems important to also systematically explore theories about society and the roles of public administration in social change.

There are people today thinking and writing about the place of critical theory in contemporary society, and some who apply critical thought in public administration. Some of this work is based in significant part on the ideas of Frankfurt school writers, and some take into account the context of postmodernism, technological advance, globalization, and the like. The time may be right for these ideas to be given greater attention in public administration. Though to lapse into passivity and pessimism is understandable, it may be hoped that part of the field's scholarship and practice will run counter to deepening one-dimensionality and the confusion about values and ends that accompanies loss of foundational certainty. As Ben Agger (2002, p. 195) writes, "meaninglessness need not thwart action if we understand that history, however devoid of millennial telos, is still available to human deliberation and design."

— 2 —

Contradiction, Utopia, and Public Administration

In 1964, in the midst of a dominant political-economic system providing an unprecedented standard of living, Herbert Marcuse's One-Dimensional Man *challenged the status quo. Marcuse argued there exists a contradiction between a life of material plenty supported by instrumental thought crowding out awareness of alternatives, and potential life options people might choose if they were free to understand them. This contradiction is evident in four areas of social practice discussed by Marcuse in several works: democracy, the "Warfare State," research, and gender. The paper relates Marcuse's analyses of these areas of practice and his utopian solutions, suggesting they may be useful for public administration theory and practice.*

Because it is a field with little inherent theoretical grounding, public administration imports theories from disciplines such as economics, business, history, philosophy, and so on. This essay fits the pattern by importing social theorist Herbert Marcuse's use of the concept *contradiction* and related ideas. Marcuse's analysis of modernist society is unusual and prescient. The premise here is that a portion of the analysis, considering the passage of four decades and modifications necessary to make it applicable today, connects with current conditions and public administration in remarkable

From *Administrative Theory & Praxis*, vol. 25, no. 2 (June 2003): 243–260. Copyright © 2003 Public Administration Theory Network. Reprinted with permission.

ways, illustrating the continuity of important theoretical matters affecting the field and yielding useful insights for public administration theory. The focus is on four areas related to contradiction—democracy, the "Warfare State," research, and gender—and Marcuse's utopian vision for social change.

Marcuse's critical thought developed over the span of his work from the 1930s through the 1970s. He became an (unintended) icon of the radical left in the 1960s, regarding political protest as a hopeful sign that resistance to the dominant economic order might be possible. Though Marcuse fits within a Hegelian-Marxist tradition, he adapted his thinking to emerging conditions. He did not give up hope for social renewal as had his Frankfurt school colleagues Max Horkheimer and Theodor Adorno, and he did not follow Jürgen Habermas in replacing labor with communication as the central feature of social analysis (Kellner, 1984, p. 91). Despite his gloomy view of conditions in society, Marcuse was a hopeful advocate of radical institutional change (p. 364). He abandoned what he considered the obsolete Marxist model of an uprising of the alienated industrial laboring class, incorporating in his analysis white-collar jobs created by the technology of the modern economy.

Marcuse drew his critical theory of society from observation of current conditions and from an Enlightenment commitment to human emancipation from repressive social systems, into a life of freedom and self-determination. As Douglas Kellner (1984, p. 365) put it, "throughout his writing there is a dialectic of the individual versus society, in which society is criticized for repressing and alienating human beings." Marcuse's early work, like that of other Frankfurt critical theorists, was shaped by grim conditions facing the laboring class and the harsh reality of Nazism.

However, Marcuse continually adapted his theoretic work to emerging conditions. When *One-Dimensional Man* was published in 1964, the world as perceived by Marcuse was that of stable liberal-capitalist democracy in its standoff with authoritarian communism. In this setting, the economic system is built on overdevelopment of natural resources, creating an excess of consumer goods. This destructive system is sustained in part by identification of external enemies and aggressive national behavior, resulting in a perpetual culture of war. Capitalism is successful in containing individual desires for change by providing workers with the necessities of life and a surplus of consumer goods, resulting in a population that, except for a radical few, is happy with the status quo. In this administered, "one-dimensional" life, people fulfill their function as producers in the economic system, kept unaware of alternatives by those with wealth and power. If meaningful social change is possible, for Marcuse it would lead to a society in which people work for self-fulfillment instead of performing boring and repetitive chores to make a living, the relationship of humans and the environment would be brought into balance, and violence and brutality would diminish.

Such broadscale analysis does not fit well into the somewhat solipsistic contemporary mood of skepticism about grand narratives, the anti-foundationalism that characterizes current epistemological thought, and the apparent victory of global capitalism. Further, on the level of perception and belief, Marcuse's vision of the world seems like a bad dream, an odd and strangely twisted version of what seems to many to be a successful and worthwhile society. Of course, that is exactly his point—the success of modernist economic social organization ensures that awareness of alternatives fades into acceptance of what is given as that which must be.

In the sections to follow, it is suggested that elements of Marcuse's critical theory of society are useful tools for understanding the present and future. The element of contradiction is the focus of this particular discussion and possible links are offered to public administration theory. Though Marcuse's work may be dismissed by some as dated, it parallels in interesting ways the thought of contemporary writers and, in its far-reaching scope, offers a new perspective on issues of current relevance.

That Marcuse's thought is useful today is not an original idea; writing in appreciation of Marcuse on what would have been his one hundredth birthday in 1998, Jürgen Habermas noted:

> Marcuse conceptualized the peculiar entwinement of the productivity of economic growth with the destructivity of its social consequences in imploring-totalizing terms, that is, with concepts that have become foreign to us. With his diagnosis Marcuse confronted us with an image of a totalitarian closed society because he believed it was necessary to introduce a vocabulary that would open clouded eyes to things that were no longer perceived at all, by casting a harsh light on familiar phenomena. (Habermas, 1998; in Kellner, 2001, p. 237)

Observing that societal conditions today make it difficult to ignore Marcuse's vision, Habermas wrote:

> No one who reads the newspaper today can deceive himself about the entwinement of productivity and destructivity. Driven by a highly efficient geopolitical competition, our governments have let themselves become entrapped in a deregulatory race to lower costs leading in the past decade to obscene profits and drastic disparities of income, deterioration of cultural infrastructures, increasing unemployment and marginalization of an increasingly

large, impoverished population. . . . The intellectual situation has changed as well. Postmodernism has disarmed the self-understanding of modernity. . . . Perhaps we need a renovated language after all, so that the pressure to conform to functional imperatives does not lead us to forget this normative viewpoint. (p. 238)

Contradiction and Containment

Contrast between opposing positions is found in literature, politics, philosophy, and so on. An important element of critical theory is a sort of contrast referred to as *contradiction*, an "opposition of forces, tendencies" (Marcuse, 1964, p. 140) in which currently accepted reality is questioned and rejected in whole or in part. From its negation a new condition or understanding emerges and after a time it, too, is questioned. Contradiction is not a static relationship between opposites, but is instead dialectical, inherently involving change, movement from one perspective to another within an idea or situation. Karl Marx adapted contradiction from the thought of Hegel, arguing that social conditions contain within themselves their own negative. In *Reason and Revolution*, Marcuse (1960, p. ix) wrote that the function of dialectical thought "is to break down the self-assurance and self-contentment of common sense, to undermine the sinister confidence in the power and language of facts, to demonstrate that unfreedom is so much at the core of things that the development of their internal contradictions leads necessarily to qualitative change: the explosion and catastrophe of the established state of affairs."

Unlike positivism, contradiction does not represent a unitary, given reality, but instead suggests that everything is in the process of change, as contradicting ideas challenge current thought. Frederick Engels (1877, pp. 3–5) described the concept in this way:

> True, so long as we consider things as at rest and lifeless, each one by itself, alongside and after each other, we do not run up against any contradictions in them. We find certain qualities which are partly common to, partly different from, and even contradictory to each other, but which in the last-mentioned case are distributed among different objects and therefore contain no contradiction within. Inside the limits of this sphere of observation we can get along on the basis of the usual, metaphysical mode of thought. But the position is quite different as soon as we consider things in their motion, their change, their life, their reciprocal influence on one another. Then we immediately become involved in contradictions. . . .
>
> Life is therefore also a contradiction which is present in things and processes themselves, and which constantly originates and resolves itself; and as soon as the contradiction ceases, life, too, comes to an end, and death steps in.

Awareness of aspects of apparent reality that are not as they could be leads to critique and thought of alternatives; this is the change process of contradiction. Marcuse takes care to distance himself from Hegel's attempt to resolve all contradictions in a unitary absolute, instead suggesting the critical reason that identifies and resolves contradictions may also be used to criticize the outcomes. Reason has been "instrumental in sustaining injustice, toil, and suffering" (Marcuse, 1941, p. xiii) in addition to promoting constructive change, so people must take responsibility for their thought and action. To think about contradictions in social conditions and to act on their knowledge, human beings must be free; thus, freedom becomes an essential element of contradiction and social change.

A brief outline of Marcuse's view of liberal-capitalist society was given above. His view begins with attention to class division and issues of power and domination in the manner of Marx, but Marcuse is a writer of the mid-twentieth century, not the nineteenth century. His analysis of modern political economy developed over the course of his career, though its most complete statement is found in *One-Dimensional Man*. Marcuse recognized that the oppressed laborers of early capitalism did not rise up to overthrow the political-economic system and that the standard of living for the largest percentage of the people in developed countries is very different from what it was a century ago. Contemporary workers are integrated into a system of production and consumption that demands their full commitment to performing the often routine and boring tasks required to make a living. There is a "progressing transfer of power from the human individual to the technical or bureaucratic apparatus" (Marcuse, 2001b, p. 65), and the system rewards conformity and compliance with material goods. Institutions of media, entertainment, education, and politics reinforce the message that production and consumption are good and the resulting environmental degradation is acceptable.

Marcuse introduces the performance principle, which helps in understanding the relationship of the individual to the workplace. The performance principle is an adaptation of Freud's reality principle (delay and/or decrease in gratification in response to external conditions) to modern, large-scale society. According to Marcuse (1955, p. 35):

> Behind the reality principle lies the fundamental fact of Ananke or scarcity (*Lebensnot*), which means that the struggle for existence takes place in a world too poor for the satisfaction of human needs without constant restraint, renunciation, delay. In other words, whatever satisfaction is possible necessitates *work*, more or less painful arrangements and undertakings for the procurement of the means for satisfying needs. For the duration of work, which

occupies practically the entire existence of the mature individual, pleasure is "suspended" and pain prevails.

However, Marcuse emphasizes that expression of the reality principle is historically determined, that is, the form it takes is in response to "a specific *organization* of scarcity" existing at a particular point in time (p. 36). This organization of scarcity is not a random happening, but is constructed intentionally, since "the *distribution* of scarcity as well as the effort of overcoming it, the mode of work, have been *imposed* on individuals—first by mere violence, subsequently by a more rational utilization of power" (p. 36). (As an example, in the history of capitalism in the United States, consider the turbulence of the transition from independent livelihood to employment in factories and other organizations, from the second half of the nineteenth century into the twentieth century, including the violence accompanying attempted suppression of the movement to organize labor.) This is not surprising, since "all civilization has been organized domination" (p. 34), which "is exercised by a particular group or individual in order to sustain and enhance itself in a privileged position" (p. 36).

In this situation, the political and economic system swallows up knowledge of alternatives, as "the world tends to become the stuff of total administration, which absorbs even the administrators" (Marcuse, 1964, p. 169). The essential characteristic of such a world is that society, people, and thought are *one-dimensional* (Kellner, 1984, pp. 234–235); that is, knowledge of contradictions has become vague or nonexistent and dialectic as an engine of social change has ceased to function. As Marcuse put it in a lecture in 1956:

> It is as though the free space which the individual has at his disposal for his psychic processes has been greatly narrowed down; it is no longer possible for something like an individual psyche with its own demands and decisions to develop; the space is occupied by public, social forces. This reduction of the relatively autonomous ego is empirically observable in people's frozen gestures, and the growing passivity of leisure-time activities, which become more and more inescapably de-privatized, centralized, universalized in the bad sense, and as such controlled. This process is the psychic correlate of the social overpowering of the opposition, the impotence of criticism, technical co-ordination, and the permanent mobilization of the collective. (in Kellner, 1984, p. 238)

Marcuse's description of society parallels Francis Fukuyama's (1992) neo-Hegelian "end of history" in its resolution of class and power contradictions within political/economic systems into a permanent condition of liberal capitalism. However, Marcuse did not think contradiction as a force for change had been eliminated; rather, it had been made invisible to the mass of people by conditioning. He called the action of controlling and obscuring contradiction, for the purpose of minimizing and suppressing dissent, *containment*. Instead of an end to ideological conflict, for Marcuse:

> in a specific sense advanced industrial culture is *more* ideological than its predecessor, inasmuch as today the ideology is in the process of production itself. . . . The productive apparatus and the goods and services which it produces "sell" or impose the social system as a whole. . . . The products indoctrinate and manipulate; they promote a false consciousness which is immune against its falsehood. . . . It is a good way of life—much better than before—and as a good way of life, it militates against qualitative change. (1964, pp. 11–12)

A parallel to Marcuse's broad social theory of containment can be found at the level of social systems such as institutions and organizations. Donald Schon describes systemic "dynamic conservatism," which "results from the workings of self-interest in those individuals who are able to see the connection between their own self-interest and the interests of the social system as a whole." Even when an individual might perceive the "non-rational character" of resistance to change, the "power of social systems over individuals" overrides individual thought, because "social systems provide for their members not only sources of livelihood, protection against outside threat and the promise of economic security, but a framework of theory, values, and related technology which enables individuals to make sense of their lives" (Schon, 1971, p. 51). Thus, when a perceived threat to current institutional or organizational practice "cannot be totally repulsed, or when it is internal and cannot be eradicated, dynamic conservatism runs to strategies of containment and isolation. Allow the threatened change a limited scope of activity and keep it bottled up" (p. 49).

One-dimensional society as described by Marcuse is not the inevitable outcome of a progressive process of human improvement, but a condition maintained through considerable effort by those who would lose the most from its dissolution. It is supported by social practices that prevent awareness of the one-dimensional nature of society and its possible alternatives, thus containing potential social change. Four such areas of practice are discussed below.

Democracy

The first area of social practice supporting containment is the nature of democracy in capitalist society. The nature of democracy as a concept, in particular the tension between direct citizen self-determination and representational governance, has always been a concern. As Rousseau put it in 1762, "The waning of patriotism, the activity of private interest, the immenseness of States, the abuse of the government have led to the invention of using deputies or representatives of the people in the nation's assemblies. . . . Sovereignty cannot be represented. . . . The English people think it is free. It greatly deceives itself; it is free only during the election of the members of Parliament. As soon as they are elected, it is a slave, it is nothing" (1978, p. 102).

The tension between direct and representational democracy is reflected in the desire of colonial-era Americans to minimize differences of status and wealth in society and in the debate between Anti-Federalists and Federalists about governmental structure (Wood, 1969). It is found in the community center movement during the Progressive era (Mattson, 1998) and in the ongoing concern in public administration about the relationship of politics and administration.

Within the context of critical social theory and the one-dimensionality of capitalist society, Marcuse regards direct citizen involvement in governance as genuine democracy. The current form of democracy, in which the "integrated, conservative majority . . . expresses its opinion, chooses between given alternatives, and thus determines policy while the decisions determining the life and death of the people are made by a ruling group beyond popular . . . control," he labels *sham-democracy* (Marcuse, 1972, p. 54).

One of several parallels to Marcuse's view of democracy within public administration scholarship can be found in Fox and Miller's (1995, p. 5) elaboration of the procedural model of democracy, which they call the "representative democratic accountability feedback loop." Though the language used and the underlying assumptions about society are quite different from those of Marcuse, Fox and Miller also characterize loop democracy as undemocratic, arguing that this form of governance, "which begins with individual preferences that are aggregated to popular will, codified by legislation, implemented by the bureaucracy, and evaluated in turn by attentive voters—lacks credibility." They give several reasons for this lack of credibility (pp. 16–17), including: "the wants and needs of the people are, by and large, manipulated" by media that are rewarded by advertisers for creating titillating sensationalism; in campaigns, image is valued over substance; public policy is shaped in part by lobbyists and political contributions; and, citizens are largely inattentive to public matters. One only needs to add the overarching conceptual framework of one-dimensional society to find the parallel to sham-democracy.

In the literature of public affairs, advocates of "deliberative democracy" hope to meliorate the antidemocractic effects of large-scale representational systems (Bohman, 1996; Yankelovich, 1991; Young, 2000). Varieties of citizen involvement techniques are suggested to improve public access to, and influence over, a policy process that has become removed from public view because of bureaucratization and/or elite control (Box, 1998; King & Stivers, 1998). Public administration discourse theorists, using critical theory, pragmatism, psychoanalytic theory, institutional and organizational analysis, and other approaches, seek ways to make public governance more democratic, less remote and alienating (Box, 2002; Farmer, 1995; Fox & Miller, 1995; King, 2000; McSwite, 1997).

Improved dialogue between citizens and public professionals may prove to be too little, too late, a fragmentary and fragile form of melioration. Sham-democracy is more complex than the matter of structures of representation, involving also problems of citizen disengagement with public affairs and the question of what purposes public administrators must serve in the one-dimensional society. If public administrators are caught between the potential for change and systemic relations of power and organizational authority, if they must be ultimately accountable to those who create, maintain, and benefit from the dominant economic order, then one action option is to avoid, to the extent possible, doing harm through needless coercion. This is part of "antiadministration," as David John Farmer (1995, 1998) has called it. Antiadministration need not exclude dialogue and constructive change, but rather would demonstrate a sensitivity to the impact of the administrative state on "private lives" (Box, 2001).

The revealed character of democracy described by Marcuse is completely different from the image commonly accepted by the public, an image consisting of simple ideas shorn of contradiction and inequity. This image collapses the complex historical story of struggle between competing ideologies and classes into a static picture painted by the winners in support of the status quo, a unitary picture in which heroic, wise, and public-regarding men created the current system, the ideal model of democratic structure and practice.

In public administration, this simplified, idealized picture is reflected in student lack of knowledge about historical development, models of citizenship, the roles of women and minorities, movements of reform, and the applicability of this context to the daily challenges of public affairs. The result is that citizens and students who may become public sector leaders are unaware of the need, much less the possibilities for, constructive social change. Public administration scholars are in a unique position to expand citizen and student knowledge beyond the given, encouraging critical thought about the role of the practitioner in society (Box & King, 2000). The unique contribution of Marcuse to the considerable body of literature in public affairs related to democracy is the characterization of one-dimensional society, including the contradiction between the ideal and the practice of democracy, and the potential for change highlighted by dialectical thought.

The Warfare State

A second area of containment of social change is the identification of external enemies and maintenance of a constant state of war. In the post–World War II period this phenomenon was described by writers such as sociologist C. Wright Mills, who called it "the permanent war economy" (Mattson, 2002, p. 61; Mills, 1958, chap. 10). According to Marcuse, maintenance of a constant state of war serves as a distraction from actual conditions in society, generates a sense of solidarity, and strengthens the economy (Kellner, 1984, p. 253), so that, "when the people, aptly stimulated by the public and private authorities, prepare for lives of total mobilization, they are sensible not only because of the present Enemy, but also because of the investment and employment possibilities in industry and entertainment" (Marcuse, 1964, p. 52). In this setting, "the society as a whole becomes a defense society" (p. 51), "which wages war or is prepared to wage war all over the world" (Marcuse, 2001b, p. 65). Writing at the height of the Vietnam War, Marcuse (2001d, p. 168) describes the "warfare government" as "a government of the representatives of the big corporations (and big labor!), a government unable (or unwilling) to halt inflation and eliminate unemployment, a government cutting down welfare and education, a government permeated with corruption, propped up by a Congress which has reduced itself to a yes-machine (after some not very serious criticism)." Citizens come to believe the logic of the Warfare State, that it is imperative to physically coerce others to do as we wish. So, "they are the ones who elect the Presidents and Vice Presidents of aggression, and their representatives increase year by year the budget of destruction" (p. 168).

During the early part of the Vietnam War and more than two decades before the fall of the Soviet Union, Marcuse recognized that communist and capitalist nations had reached an uneasy accommodation. In his view, the enemy had become localized wars of national liberation, not because they threatened the capitalist countries' access to resources or cheap labor, but because they represented:

41

the danger of a subversion of the established hierarchy of master and servant, top and bottom, a hierarchy that has created and sustained the have-nations, capitalist and communist. There is a very primitive, very elemental threat of subversion—a slave revolt rather than a revolution, and precisely for this reason more dangerous to societies that are capable of containing or defeating revolutions. For the slaves are everywhere and countless, and they have indeed nothing to lose but their chains. (Marcuse, 2001b, pp. 66–67)

The world has changed since Marcuse wrote, and communism is no longer a serious threat. However, this only makes his words seem more powerful today—an extended review of world conditions as this is being written at the end of 2002 is not necessary for readers to grasp the uncanny parallel. To restate a bit of Habermas from above, "no one who reads the newspaper today can deceive himself about the entwinement of productivity and destructivity." Many Americans remember President Bush's exhortation to Americans in the period immediately following the terrorist attacks of September 11, 2001. As his government geared up to "smoke" the evil ones out of their caves and catch them "dead or alive," Americans were urged to go out and shop, to consume as much as we could to help keep the economy healthy. (Some of us are of an age to have grown up with cowboy radio and television shows and films, but—I note with some relief—most of us have not carried that language into our adult lives.)

Recently, as his administration adopted a policy of preemptive military strikes against countries that might harbor terrorists or build "weapons of mass destruction," President Bush (who lacks the skill or desire, or both, to mask economic motivation) declared that America was justified in doing so because of the threat to the U.S. economy. These ideas seem to create a sense of national unity, one that Marcuse (2001c, p. 157) anticipated as he wrote that "the leaders still deliver the goods (and periodically, the bodies of the enemies who threaten the delivery of those goods)."

The Warfare State seems a bit removed from public administration teaching and practice, since few of us can directly affect events at this level. However, public administration students and the citizens they serve can be thought of as carriers of a self-deceptive cultural narrative (Betsworth, 1990) that perpetuates the Warfare State. Many Americans have in some measure accepted the logic of constant defense buildup and intervention in the affairs of other nations without knowing much if anything about elements of their national history that contradict this condition. This is not a matter of whether a nation should defend itself in time of crisis, but of how a people relate to the world and their place in it. It may be argued that an evangelical, interventionist model of international behavior, one that assumes a responsibility to shape other nations and peoples in one's own image

(Betsworth, 1990, chap. 5), spills over into intranational affairs and attitudes as well.

The idea that violence and coercion are appropriate means toward the end of shaping the thought and action of others need not go unchallenged. Media commentators are now raising questions about the role of America in the world. This is useful, but Marcuse's work goes beyond current events, to the nature of the society that promotes and supports the actions in question, a society Marcuse believed to be based on one-dimensional suppression of alternatives to current patterns of labor, economics, environmental degradation, power, and international domination.

Research

A third area of societal practice supporting containment of change is a particular variety of academic research. Marcuse's perspective is based on Hegelian contradiction and dialectic that allow the thinker to move beyond the given knowledge of sense experience, subjecting it to critical reason that identifies its negative elements and explores possibilities for change. To contain and neutralize such critique, common sense and positivism "induces thought to be satisfied with the facts, to renounce any transgression beyond them, and to bow to the given state of affairs" (Marcuse, 1941, p. 27). We may argue about what this means for the practice of public administration, since many citizens and elected officials would prefer public professionals to restrict their thought and action to the given, the present, the accepted. This is the value-fact, politics-administration divide that, though claimed by some academicians to be long dead, is alive and well in the value assumptions and expectations of the public. Thus, it may be prudent for a practitioner—even one inclined to critically examine what is, with intent to imagine what could be—to suppress critical thinking in the interest of personal career safety.

It might be thought that people whose profession is oriented toward searching for knowledge rather than applying it, that is, academicians, would feel, if not duty bound to critically examine the apparent, the given, then at least curious about what might result from such an examination. However, the "scientific" conception of the study of human affairs "cancels from the domain of knowledge everything that may not yet be a fact" (p. 113), and academicians are pressured to conform to norms of inquiry that exclude rationalistic, ideological speculation, thereby assuring colleagues they are legitimate members of the community of inquiry. As a result, "the difference between the destination of mankind and its present course"

(Horkheimer, 1947, p. 53) is suppressed, ignored, in favor of an instrumental version of reason that "has become completely harnessed to the social process. Its operational value, its role in the domination of men and nature, has been made the sole criterion" (p. 21).

Marcuse calls the use of research to solidify one-dimensional knowledge the *research of total administration*. Few would deny the need for description, measurement and quantification in social science. The question is not whether they are needed, but whether their accompanying epistemological paradigm should be normatively preferred to the exclusion of other perspectives. This is a matter of the purposes of scholarly inquiry. When the purpose is "therapeutic," isolating the object of research from the characteristics of the surrounding society in "the service of exploring and improving the existing social conditions," then "if the given form of society is and remains the ultimate frame of reference for theory and practice, there is nothing wrong with this sort of sociology and psychology. It is more human and more productive to have good labor-management relations than bad ones, to have pleasant rather than unpleasant working conditions, to have harmony rather than conflict between the desires of the customers and the needs of business and politics" (Marcuse, 1964, p. 107).

For scholars in the social sciences, and particularly in a field with applied usefulness such as public administration, the weight of the expectation to produce research of value to the economic system is substantial. It can be reinforced in practical and immediate ways through processes of peer review of research and standards for tenure, promotion, and increases in compensation. This expectation serves as an implementation vehicle for fashionable societal attitudes about education, which is "increasingly functional: oriented on the jobs to be had and to be done: rewarded service to the establishment" (Marcuse, 2001d, p. 169).

Today, practice and research in public administration seem to be oriented as much as ever toward economic efficiency and quantification, to the exclusion of other values (such as duty of public service, fostering democratic discourse, social equity). The broad societal context is that of economic globalization and standardization to an extent Marcuse could not have foreseen, though he would hardly have been surprised. In this context, scholarly writing that does not conform to the one-dimensional epistemology of liberal capitalism is likely to be surrounded, attacked, and contained before it can spread. The initial attack is often on grounds that such writing is not "empirical," once a word with broad meaning that has been whittled down to fit a one-dimensional view of research, exemplified by "the fine little mill of The Statistical Ritual" (Mills, 1959, p. 72).

The reality to be contained is that phenomena observed by researchers are nested in broader historical and social contexts that are either constantly changing or have within them the potential to change under critical examination. This context and its potential for change may influence, and be influenced by, the phenomenon under observation. To label the broader context of research irrelevant or inapplicable is a misunderstanding of what is empirical, potentially resulting in flawed, incomplete knowledge, a "false concreteness" (Marcuse, 1964, pp. 106–107).

Gender

The fourth and last area of social practice to be discussed consists of the dominance of masculine qualities in society. According to Kellner (1984, pp. 340–341), Marcuse regarded "aggression, competition, and repression" of "creative receptivity" as characteristics of "the dominant masculine values and the capitalist performance principle," which drives people to perform repetitive, self-destructive labor. Marcuse believed the technology of advanced capitalism was being used to reinforce wasteful production of multiple consumer goods instead of allowing people time and freedom to choose their work in keeping with their interests and self-development. Mobilization of resources and societal institutions to create and maintain aggressive, competitive productivity spills over into government and politics, so that "technological rationality operates as political rationality" (Marcuse, 2001a, p. 47). In contrast to earlier periods of history, modern society has been successful "in integrating and reconciling antagonistic groups and interests: bipartisan policy, acceptance of the national purpose, co-operation of business and labor testify to this achievement." Though there are occasional conflicts, overall:

> One of the accomplishments of advanced industrial civilization is the nonterroristic, democratic decline of freedom—the efficient, smooth, reasonable unfreedom which seems to have its roots in technical progress itself. What could be more rational than the suppression of individual autonomy in the mechanization and standardization of socially necessary but painful performances, the concentration of private enterprises in more effective and more productive corporations, the regulation of free competition among unequally equipped economic subjects, the curtailment of prerogatives and national sovereignties which impede the international organization of resources. (Marcuse, 2001a, p. 37)

[It might be interesting to interject a brief historical digression, specifically a bit of Alexis de Tocqueville's commentary on America in the early nineteenth century. It presents a startling parallel to Marcuse's analysis of the intertwining of economics and politics in the later twentieth century. As he thought ahead into the distant future, Tocqueville (1969, p. 692) wondered whether America might not evolve to the point that:

> Having thus taken each citizen in turn in its powerful grasp and shaped him to its will, government then extends its embrace to include the whole of society. It covers the whole of social life with a network of petty, complicated rules that are both minute and uniform, through which even men of the greatest originality and the most vigorous temperament cannot force their heads above the crowd. It does not break men's will, but softens, bends, and guides it; it seldom enjoins, but often inhibits, action; it does not destroy anything, but prevents much being born; it is not at all tyrannical, but it hinders, restrains, enervates, stifles, and stultifies so much that in the end each nation is no more than a flock of timid and hardworking animals with the government as its shepherd.]

Writing during the beginning of the modern women's liberation movement, Marcuse (2001d, p. 182) thought "the negation of the values and goals of the male-dominated patriarchal society is also the negation of the values and goals of capitalism—and this on the physiological, instinctual level of the individual." Marcuse noted he had been criticized for accepting a sexist view of women by ascribing to them qualities such as tenderness or softness that are "actually socially determined," but he preferred to avoid the controversy over whether certain human characteristics are the result of nature or society. Creative receptivity and softness may have been forced on women by the historical development of capitalism and their separation from the workplace (though this separation can be traced at least to the ancient Greeks; see Elshtain, 1981).

For Marcuse (2001d, p. 182), however, the point regarding these characteristics is that "they can be put to political, social use. . . . The goal is to free those qualities (male and female) which pertain to a better society, a society without sexual and other exploitation—regardless of whether these qualities are physiologically or socially determined." The potential is for "the promise of peace, of joy, of the end of violence" (Marcuse, 1972, p. 77). The dialectical process between patriarchal capitalist society and the "female image" could result in a "counter-force, which may still become one of the gravediggers of patriarchal society" (p. 78).

The significance for public administration of a change in emphasis from dominant reliance on what Marcuse describes as masculine values, to a more balanced mixture of feminine and masculine values, could be significant. Practice could be affected in many areas, including the structures and management of organizations, agency stance in relation to politics and the private sector, and discourse processes with citizens. Academicians might choose to teach technical, instrumental skills within a broader human context, giving students a richer, more sophisticated conceptual basis for their work. They might also critically examine their research to understand what societal values and interests it serves.

Refusal and Utopia

This discussion has focused on only a few areas of Marcuse's thought, chosen for their possible relation to public administration theory. It is heady stuff, surprising in the way radical leftist thought of the 1940s through 1970s connects to, explains, and suggests ways to address the current situation. It can be difficult to hear, in part because it requires setting aside contemporary aversion to metanarrative and broad social theory, and in part because Marcuse may be right: we are increasingly closed off to alternatives as one-dimensional thinking becomes the norm.

Marcuse was pleased at the social resistance among students and intellectuals in the 1960s and 1970s. Though he did not think it sufficient to cause much change, he hoped it might in the long term build toward something more significant. He thought change, because of the nature of the current society, would have to take place as a "determinate negation," in a *break* with the present (Marcuse, 1970, p. 76). One way people could express their disapproval of present conditions is the *Great Refusal*, in which people refuse to participate in much of what modern society offers and requires. This is not a call to a collective social movement, but the withdrawal of individuals from society in the interest of a "pacified existence," with human qualities that now

> seem asocial and unpatriotic—qualities such as the refusal of all toughness, togetherness, and brutality; disobedience to the tyranny of the majority; profession of fear and weakness (the most rational reaction to this society!); a sensitive intelligence sickened by that which is being perpetrated; the commitment to the feeble and ridiculed actions of protest and refusal. These expressions of humanity, too, will be marred by necessary compromise—by the need to cover oneself, to be capable of cheating the cheaters, and to live and think in spite of them. (Marcuse, 1964, pp. 242–243)

This is not a hopeful vision, but given Marcuse's analysis of societal conditions, the likelihood of organized, collective change seemed remote and an individual turning away appeared to be what remained. At other times Marcuse (1969, p. 89) could be more optimistic, envisioning spontaneous action by "small groups, widely diffused, with a high degree of autonomy, mobility, flexibility." These groups would work toward a utopian vision "in which the stupefying, enervating, pseudo-automatic jobs of capitalist progress would be abolished" (p. 21), and their members would demonstrate a sensitivity to "the difference between calm and noise, tenderness and brutality, intelligence and stupidity, joy and fun, and it would correlate this distinction with that between freedom and servitude" (p. 91). The utopian end product of these change efforts Marcuse (in Kellner, 1984, p. 322) called *libertarian socialism*, to distinguish it from the statist socialism of the twentieth century, and to emphasize human freedom. The idea of decentralized discourse and action toward a utopian future finds parallels within the history and practice of public administration in, for example, aspects of the Progressive era, the "new public administration" of the 1960s and 1970s, and current models of public discourse and citizen self-governance.

Though Marcuse's language may make his ideas seem removed from the practice and theory of public administration, the literature of the field often parallels Marcuse, sometimes reaching conclusions not unlike his though the underlying assumptions about knowledge and the nature of society may differ. Forms of democratic practice, the position of the citizen in relation to government, the purposes of governmental action, the contrast between administrative values of men and women, the nature of academic research, and alternative responses to social conditions are all addressed in some form in public administration. Like the rest of life, public administration is surrounded by contradictions, by practices (theory in use) that differ from what we want to believe are the purposes of government (espoused theory). An overarching contradiction affecting theory and practice is that between public service/public interest and government as reflection of the interests of the market.

Public administration academicians and practitioners may be aware, if sometimes in fragmentary and uncertain ways, of the contradictions in their professional surroundings and of the action alternatives available to them. To deny or ignore the contradictions, turn away from social conditions in refusal, or work toward meaningful social change are choices dependent on time, circumstance, and personal preference. If nothing else, Marcuse's ideas invite us to evaluate our social, political, economic, and physical environments and our relation to them.

— 3 —

The "T"ruth is Elsewhere: Critical History

This essay begins by deconstructing the basic question of how the present is defined in traditional historical explanation or analysis. It is our contention that to "rewrite" the present, one must be critical, examining the assumptions and methods behind historical "data" to identify what might be missed—whose stories are silenced—when theorists rely upon only the "great stories" of past events or "great men," and to reveal metanarratives of history that support dominant regimes, hegemonies, and power structures. We then examine theoretical approaches to the use of theory, pointing out examples relevant to public administration.

> Until the lions have their historians, tales of hunting will always glorify the hunter.
> —*Old African proverb*

> . . . we need it [history] for life and action, not for a comfortable turning away from life and action or merely for glossing over the egotistical life and the cowardly bad act.

> It requires a great deal of power to be able to live and to forget just how much life and being unjust are one and the same.
> —*F.W. Nietzsche,* On the Use and Abuse of History for Life, 1873

With Cheryl Simrell King, from *Administrative Theory & Praxis*, vol. 22, no. 4 (December 2000): 751–771. Copyright © 2000 Public Administration Theory Network. Reprinted with permission.

In this essay, we start by deconstructing the basic question of how the present is defined in traditional historical explanation or analysis. In doing so, the epistemological and ontological assumptions of history, as it is traditionally defined, must be examined. As with other social science disciplines, the discipline of history has undergone a radical transformation in the last thirty years—the positivist, social scientific methods rigorously adopted during what we in public administration understand as the Progressive era have been interrogated and laid bare. At the same time that historical methodological approaches, and the ontological assumptions within, have been questioned, ironically, historicization has been adopted as a "new" method in the social sciences (including public administration). As Berkhofer (1995, p. i) states, "Poststructuralist and postmodernist theories question the possibility of writing history at the very same time that such historicization has become a way of grounding literary studies and the social sciences. That historicization is considered *so* vital by some scholars just when its whole approach to representing the past *is* being challenged by others poses a paradox." This paradox challenges scholars of history and should challenge any scholar who chooses to use history as a method of writing, particularly one who claims to be using history to "rewrite" the present.

It is our contention that to "rewrite" the present, one must, necessarily, be critical. We use the term *critical* here in two ways:

1. To critically analyze the assumptions and methods used when relying on historical "data," in order to identify what might be missed—whose stories are silenced—when theorists rely upon only the "great stories" of the past or only the stories of "great men." When we look beyond the great stories, what is exposed? What is discovered when the analytical tools of historians or of other social scientists adopting historical methods are turned on the history of "everyday life" and everyday people as a substitute for a tradition of "historiography that has largely excluded 'everyday life' from its purview" (Ludtke, 1995, p. 1)?
2. To reveal metanarratives of history as supporting dominant regimes, hegemonies, and power structures. Once this is recognized, there is a short distance between being critical of traditional historical explanation and critical theory, particularly critical theory as a historical/theoretical structure.

In the first part of this essay, we address the deconstruction of traditional historical analysis. In the second section, we discuss aspects of critical theory relevant to the study of history in public administration. Further, explicitly rejecting the ideological and epistemological etiquette of theoretical boundaries, we draw on scholars representing critical, postmodern, and pragmatic theory to offer the argument that reading, and writing, critical history are important to public administration.

Deconstructing History

The discipline of history is not immune to the epistemological revolutions of the last few decades that have brought into question the foundational values of social science disciplines. As in other disciplines, history has been accused of being saddled with the excesses of "science." In traditional historical analysis, as in other social sciences, as long as one uses established standards of "rigorous methods" and "argumentative" presentation, one is practicing good, objective historical analysis. Traditional historical analysis, usually involving "large scale contours" and "big patterns" (Ludtke, 1995, p. 10), investigates macrotheory and macroconcepts. As such, like other foundational social science theory, historical analysis has tended to be universalizing grand theory. Recent linguistic, interpretative, and rhetorical intellectual "turns" have made theorists aware of the importance of language, interpretation, and meaning to human understanding and, therefore, the importance of language, interpretation, and meaning to understanding humans. Our methodological stances, therefore, cannot objectively separate "data" or "historical texts" from their linguistic, interpretative, and rhetorical contexts. Methodologies and knowledge in the social sciences are not universal and timeless. They are socially and culturally constituted and, therefore, historically specific rather than historically universal. History, then, is perhaps even more susceptible to intellectual critique than other disciplines because it expressly tries to write our present based upon the past. To do so without contextualizing the past in its linguistic, interpretative, and rhetorical context is to write a past/present that is significantly distorted on a number of levels.

These distortions show up in history in a number of ways, much in the same way they show up in other social sciences. One distortion that readers will find familiar is the question of whose "story" is being told in "history?" In the desire to make history a value-free science, the discipline of history acted for years in denial of the "gendered," "classed," and "raced" nature of the work. Although historians' personal lives may very well be influenced by gender, race, and class, their methodology, ostensibly, allowed them to arrive as "close as humanly possible to an ungendered [unraced and unclassed] historical truth" (Smith, 1998, p. 1). According to the dogma, only "bad" (nonobjective) history would have a gendered, raced, or classed version of the past that was in opposition to accepted evidence. Changes in the profession brought on by the intellectual turns shifted the thinking in the field, but only partially, as Smith (pp. 1–2) explains:

> Changes in the profession since the early 1970s have been based on these beliefs. Trained in scientific methods, historians of both women and people of color have assumed that their scholarship would eventually fit into the field of history as a whole. Their findings fill out the picture, making scholarship of the past finally truthful . . . The profession's rationality and fairness would ultimately allow the findings of women's history and the accomplishments of women historians their full influence and dignity in the academy. When a prominent social historian announced that historical research about women had gone far enough and should stop, it was in the belief that history's claims to lack of bias could be vitiated by an excess of such information. The history of women and blacks, it was said, would politicize the field. Or these subdisciplines could undermine the truth value of real history by exposing it to influences outside professional standards for what was important.

Once distortions are exposed, there is no guarantee that the new knowledge is accepted as legitimate and usable. This stems, in part, from another significant distortion in our perceptions of the present based upon the past—how history acts as a metanarrative structure or force. History provides important ballast for the received values of a culture or a society. As such, it serves the function of promulgating the myths and structures of a culture or society. Although history believes itself to be focusing on material "reality," behavior is shaped not so much by material or "real" conditions as it is by our image of our conditions—by our perceptions rather than by what is "real." A woman is poor only if she perceives herself as such, regardless of whether she fits within some analytical category of "poor" as measured by something we call "real income." Our perceptions, social relations, and the historical transformation of both take place within value systems that form our boundaries, our limits, and set the terms of possible transgressions. These value systems, according to Duby (1985, p. 154) tend to have the following characteristics:

1. They serve a globalizing function—they claim to offer an overall representation of society, its past, present, and future. Thus, they form our ideas of the social and the individual.
2. In addition, they serve a deforming function. By highlighting some things, they obscure others all in service of particular interests. There is both light and shadow.

3. Multiple systems exist at one time and compete with one another.
4. The systems stabilize—both those systems that guard the privileges of the ruling class and those inverted (shadow) systems that invert, but reflect, the ruling class systems—one is not possible without the other. As a result, systems tend toward conservation—toward conserving the status quo.
5. The systems are visionary—in cultures that have a history, all ideological systems are based on a vision of that history—a projected future in which society will be closer to perfection is based on the memory, objective or mythical, of the past.

As a result of their globalizing, deforming, competing, stabilizing, and visionary components, historical systems focus on telling the "great story" or the story of "great men," and they distort or do not tell stories of everyday life and everyday people. Traditional historical systems of values do so, in part, to ensure that the dominant systems remain stable. Those who are interested in destabilizing historical systems focus their critique on these five functions in the attempt to show how history and historical systems continue to perpetuate the myths that keep our systems running "efficiently" and out of bounds for critique.

Western historical scholars believe that history is a mirror, reflecting back to us the "truth" about ourselves. Held up to the past, the mirror reflects exactly back to us the events of the past. How we see ourselves is determined by the images projected back to us in that mirror—who we are, how we live, what we value, how we govern—all are constituted by what is reflected back to us. If those images are consonant with our sense of self, then we dare not doubt those images (or question their "objectivity"), especially if we are of the dominant group. When that mirror is held in such a way that what is reflected threatens dominant ideologies, people will refuse to look into the mirror.

For example, an acquaintance recently remarked upon the "crazies in Seattle making a fuss for no reason" at the 1999 World Trade Organization meeting. When it was noted that they were making "a fuss," among other things, about the effects of corporate globalization on the environment and the potential future effects of exporting American lifestyles to other, highly populated countries, he readily agreed that the issues were problematic. The media and dominant value systems of the United States are set up to cast into light "troublesome" aspects of alternative visions of living while the important message is cast into shadow. To bring to light the important message (we cannot all continue to exploit and consume with apparent unending abandon) is to draw into question the basic foundations upon which the consumption economy is built. The threat that we will stop "behaving" in ways that are needed to keep the systems flourishing must remain in the shadow. If we were behaving according to the scripts defined for us, we would respond to our acquaintance in a way that would affirm the dominant messages (these people are crazy) instead of refusing to accept what is packaged to be common knowledge (globalization is good—it makes more opportunity for all!). Indeed, it may be easier to be a "system-affirmer" than it is to be a "system-refuser" (Farmer, 2000a). David John Farmer, drawing on Herbert Marcuse's great refusal, "a refusal that seems the more unreasonable the more the established system develops its productivity and alleviates the burdens of life" (Marcuse, 1964; in Farmer, 2000a, p. 644), outlines the various ways public administrators (theorists and practitioners alike) can affirm (speaking from power) or refuse (speaking to power) systems. History, as it is traditionally defined, serves as a "systems-affirmer." What we would like to see is historical analysis that serves as a "systems-refuser."

Some of our best postmodern theorists have paved the way for scholars who are interested in historical analysis evolving into a systems-refuser. For example, Michel Foucault redefined the notion of history by destabilizing or decentering the "great story" approach to history to show how historical knowing as defined by "great stories" or "great men" is an effort to control the discontinuities of life and to inhibit change. Foucault writes his histories of the present not to write the present as a mirror of the past, but to confront us with "the fragmentation, the instability, that conventional historical narratives often conceal. In seeing the instability, the shifting ground on which we stand, we can begin to think otherwise, to imagine that our pasts do not necessarily lead to a future that will validate some meaning and direction in our lives or culture" (Roth, 1995, p. 5). Richard Rorty also seeks to destabilize history, but does so from a different perspective than Foucault's. Foucault operates as if history is actually discontinuous. Rorty, on the other hand, sees history as something that can be narrated either to support an emphasis on discontinuity and fragmentation or to support an emphasis on continuity and wholeness, so that what matters is what one does with history (Roth, 1995, p. 5).

Redefining/Rediscovering History

Indeed, what matters is what one does with history. Although the discipline of history struggles with how to define itself methodologically such that distortions are minimized and the field does not become "politicized," ironically many other social science and literary disciplines have embraced historicization as a "new" methodological tool. Berkhofer (1995, p. 2) asks: "With the recent announcement of a 'historic turn,' have the human sciences come full circle to the traditional starting point of historians?" Roth (1995, p. 2) takes the question one step further:

> By the early 1980s, historical consciousness was seen by many as an ineffective, ideological, and unsophisticated mode of apprehending the world. Within the discipline of history . . . a crisis of confidence had shaken many of the most theoretically minded practitioners, as it became unclear what contribution the organized study of the past could make to the conversation of our culture. By the early 1990s much had changed. Scholars in a variety of fields were turning to the historical again as an area from which they could learn lessons essential to their disciplines (or to their attacks on their disciplines) . . . [However,] despite the increased interest in historical studies or in cultural studies with a historical dimension, questions about the basic value of historical consciousness or historical knowing remain open and vital.

Although American public administration has always relied upon historical analysis as a methodological tool (we can never get too far from our foundational documents, for example the *Federalist Papers,* the Constitution, Wilson's essay, and the Friedrich/Finer debate), historicization as an intellectual tool has recently enjoyed a renaissance of sorts. Examples include John Rohr's (1986) analysis of the "regime values" of the founding fathers, the May/June 1993 Spicer and Terry symposium on legitimacy in *Public Administration Review,* and extend to myriad articles and conference panels of the last few years that examine public administration principles and assumptions historically. Both mainstream and alternative public administration theory communities are embracing historical analysis. The question for us, however, is the degree to which scholars are critical of historical method and whether they approach history from the standpoint of elements of critical theory.

Camilla Stivers (1993) is one of the first public administration scholars to draw our attention to the limitations of historical methods—to the way historical methods shine light on some aspects of our history while casting others into shadow. In her recent book, she quotes a passage from a little known work by John Gaus (1930, cited in Stivers, 2000a, p. 2), in which he called for a "usable past" for public administration, emerging from historical "aspects . . . which now lie buried." She looks for the buried aspects in her historical analysis of the fields of public administration (bureau men) and social work (settlement women) during the Progressive era that investigates the "broader historical, intellectual, and gender dynamics that show how factors that shaped one field also influenced and were shaped by forces at work in other areas" (p. 2).

In her earlier critique of Spicer and Terry's constitutional arguments, Stivers (1993) showed how their reliance upon rational analysis (their comments on slavery notwithstanding) failed to take into account how "certain individuals and groups gained by the terms of this document and others (such as non-property owners, African-Americans, and women of all races and classes) came up short" (p. 256). She continues:

> By encouraging us to see the framers' decisions as logical, Spicer and Terry perpetuate the idea that no moral dilemmas inhabit the Constitution and, ironically, romanticize the framers by characterizing as rational their all-too-human propensity to let their own material interests shape their notion of "higher" aims. The point is that the founders could have chosen otherwise. They could have—and in some ways did—act out of something other than self-interest. As Vaclav Havel has reminded us, the greatest threat to human freedom is not the classic dictator but the phenomenon of impersonal power: power that is rooted in apparently neutral and objective logic. (p. 257)

Certainly, public administration needs more scholarship like Stivers's. In addition, we need scholarship that seeks to recover a "usable past" that consciously reflects a recognition of the power of historical scholarship to form, deform, and stabilize regimes, epistemes, and metanarratives that keep us from interrogating the received views of power in our culture. One way of recovering a usable past is through critical theory.

Recoverable Elements

Some scholarship in public administration and in fields that contribute to public administration thought contains elements of critical theory, but we may not think of it that way. Instead, we often expect critical theory to be complex and "heavy," with an unmasking of the true nature of society so that people shed false consciousness (they are enlightened), then take action that frees them from oppression (they are emancipated) (Geuss, 1981, pp. 1–2). This "Frankfurt" view has been modified by the "second generation" communicative approach of Jürgen Habermas. However, Habermas's work also involves a search for emancipation from some of the conditions of modern, rationalized society, in which the instrumental rationality of economic and administrative systems penetrates and alters the "lifeworld" of culture, society, and personality, oppressing free choice and discourse (Alway, 1995, pp. 99–127).

Critical theory has only a small audience in public administration today, in part because public administration is an applied professional field, and in part because critical theory offers broad narratives about oppression within capitalist society and the need for emancipation of whole classes of people, allowing them to realize their full human potential. Such an all-inclusive theoretical system makes it difficult to accept and use critical theory in a time of competing views on research and politics, skepticism about grand narratives such as elite domination or class consciousness, and the triumph of Western liberal-capitalist economic and political systems.

It is not our purpose to "rehabilitate" critical theory or to push it aside as failed dogma. Rather, we seek to recover core elements of critical thought that are useful for contemporary public administration, with particular attention to the value of critical thought in understanding the history of the field and the broader societal context. In so doing, we cross the boundaries of theoretical categories such as critical theory and pragmatism, modernism and postmodernism. This willingness to borrow "whatever works" will upset readers who prefer conceptual orderliness, but we are more interested in useful results than with internal consistency and try to be sensitive to the difficulties raised by eclecticism.

In outline, the sections below address some primary themes in critical theory, the condition of radical and reformist thought today, and the purposes of critical scholarly examination of administrative history, with examples of relevant literature.

Emancipation

Critical theory of the 1920s and 1930s retained the idea that the working class had the potential to rise up against capitalist exploitation, but in the post–World War II era it was clear this potential, if it ever existed, had been lost. For critical theorists, late capitalist society, with its bureaucratization, technical-instrumental reason, mass production, advertising media, and separation of work from leisure had become so pervasive that people no longer could think of any other way of being. Critical theorists believed that people were lulled into acceptance of their roles as units of production and kept satisfied with consumer goods so that social change was "contained," as Marcuse put it. The basic needs of most people in developed countries were met, wasteful overproduction of bountiful consumer goods encouraged people to accept the administered rationality of the capitalist state, and alternatives became unreal and irrational. In this setting, "domination functions as administration," so that "the administered life becomes the good life of the whole" (Marcuse, 1964, p. 255). This is the condition Marcuse called "The Happy Consciousness—the belief that the real is rational and the system delivers the goods" (p. 84).

Ben Agger (1992, p. 233) describes Theodor Adorno as having lost all hope for a critical, revolutionary subject (people ready for "revolution"), because "the subject was so damaged, with no prepolitical potential, that its thought and speech were but reflexes of the dominant ideology and discourse." During the countercultural movement of the 1960s and 1970s, Marcuse found some grounds for optimism in the radicalism of young people (Kellner, 1984), but the gloomy nature of his overall assessment of modern society in *One-Dimensional Man* (1964) cannot be mistaken. In this situation, all that is left to the person who does not accept the administered society is the "politically impotent . . . absolute refusal," which seems increasingly unreasonable "the more the established system develops its productivity and alleviates the burden of life." Critical theory cannot envision a better future, because it "possesses no concepts which could bridge the gap between the present and its future" (Marcuse, 1964, p. 257). Thus critical theory can do little more than offer critique, as, "holding no promise and showing no success, it remains negative" (p. 257).

To this point, critical theory had offered a materialist analysis of modern technological society and its mass production as the medium of oppression and domination. With the work of Habermas, attention shifted to analysis of the ways language and discourse settings can facilitate or mitigate unequal power relationships. Agger (1992, p. 182) calls this turn from broad critique of the institutions of capitalism to a narrower focus on communication "the splitting of critical theory." In Agger's narrative, "Habermas wants to restore to people the capacity to reason that has been negated by capitalist ideology, which transforms them into passive consumers of dominant political and economic wisdom as well as commodities" (p. 183). This restoration would not overturn the extant political economy, but reform it so that economic and administrative systems would not overpower the "lifeworld" of culture, society, and personality to the extent they do today. Agger views this as a narrower form of radicalism than that of earlier critical theorists, an instrumental approach that would "aim at certain piecemeal goals, such as the democratization and economic leveling of the capitalist welfare state" (p. 185). This does not go as far as the radicalism of Marcuse, who according to Agger would seek full emancipation and reunification of the spheres of work and private life "in the context of a cooperative community of coequal producers" (p. 184).

Not all critical theorists accept the view that critical theory, to be vital and popular in "postmodern" times, must shed its revolutionary intent. From a feminist perspective, Teresa Ebert (1996, p. 3) argues against what she identifies as the trend away from concern with material conditions in society (economic, institutional, systemic), a trend that emphasizes "poststructuralist assumptions about linguistic play, difference, and the priority of discourse." Ebert believes that "plurality, multiculturalism, multiplicity, and complexity have frequently been deployed to silence, suppress, occlude, and marginalize other positions and to suppress a fundamental or radical diversity: the differences of the social division of labor, of class antagonisms and the revolutionary struggle to overthrow the existing exploitative social relations" (p. 43).

Both revolutionary and incremental varieties of critical theory are challenged by postmodernism. Critical and postmodern thought find much agreement on critique of objectivity, science, and society, but postmodernists question critical theory's apparent belief in universal truth and totalizing visions of emancipation that ignore the local, everyday aspects of life (Rosenau, 1992, p. 14). Moving to protect critical theory from this challenge, Agger (1992, p. 238) would abandon strict adherence to dogmatic forms of thought, claiming "'critical theory' is not a school but the way we choose to oppose inhumanity in different songs of joy." To achieve this, critical theory would need to broaden beyond critique of "damaged life," so it may engage "contemporary issues of theory and practice and new social movements" (p. 196).

For Ebert, as for Agger, much postmodern thought serves to make social change impossible. Society becomes "an unending present of infinite striving over differences." It "valorizes the permanence of class conflict—and thus its own class privilege—in its claims for the necessity of unending antagonism: the permanence and inevitability of capitalism" (Ebert, 1996, p. 231). Ebert counters this with her belief that "emancipation—as the historically specific project of freeing people from the exploitation of the relations of production in capitalism—is neither unrealizable nor impossible" (p. 231).

Social Hope

This brings us to a discussion of what sort of social change can or should be envisioned, sought after within the contemporary context. Clearly, those who view contemporary society as oppressive and one-dimensional will differ on desired outcomes with those who view it as needing modification rather than a complete overhaul. Be that as it may, few people in the developed world think there is much potential for revolutionary change in the social order in the short term, if ever. In this setting, the task becomes understanding what potential for change exists and for what normative purposes. A good place to begin would be to examine how people view their world. Raymond Geuss (1981, p. 83) identifies "four quite different initial states" of awareness in the general population about the issues that also concern critical theorists:

1. Agents are suffering and know what social institution or arrangement is the cause.
2. Agents know that they are suffering, but either do not know what the cause is or have a false theory about the cause.
3. Agents are apparently content, but analysis of their behavior shows them to be suffering from hidden frustration of which they are not aware.
4. Agents are actually content, but only because they have been prevented from developing certain desires which in the "normal" course of things they would have developed, and which cannot be satisfied within the framework of the present social order.

People are not uniform in relation to these four initial states. Marcuse's characterization of a "one-dimensional," technical-rational society may hold some validity in the aggregate, though it assumes there are alternatives people might find preferable if they knew about them. Many scholars do not make that assumption and are content to work within the current societal-economic structure. Even if one accepts Marcuse's characterization of existing society and the desirability of seeking alternatives, it would be inappropriate to assume that all people in a community, region, nation, or collection of nations are alike in knowledge of their situation or preferences for social change.

Many or most people in developed countries are fully integrated into the dominant capitalist-consumerist culture and many in developing countries strive to be. It is not a failure of commitment to social betterment to acknowledge the difficulty of convincing masses of people that the only system they trust to offer material comfort and a measure of liberty is somehow illusory, oppressive, and defective. However, this is not to deny the existence of significant dissatisfaction with contemporary society and that it takes many forms. Using groups and movements as shorthand to identify a few examples, we could include people who draw their values from religion, resistance to government (militias, libertarianism), back-to-the-land philosophy, "voluntary simplicity," the search for racial, gender, economic, and other forms of social justice, communitarianism, and so on. Some people involved in these movements or bodies of thought probably fit within Geuss's category 1 and believe they can expand awareness in the general population so that people in categories 2–4 can come to share their understanding.

Marcuse, recognizing the failure of workers to serve as a revolutionary class, drew some consolation from the activities of radical youth as a possible precursor to widespread revolutionary consciousness, but the point here is not a search for an entire class of people ready to overthrow the existing order. Instead, it is to suggest that awareness of the damaging effects of late-modern/postmodern society, and the desire for change, is neither absent nor equally distributed in populations. This awareness and desire may not be sufficient to initiate wholesale radical change, but it may be adequate to the task of making "proposals for specific changes in social arrangements—in laws, company regulations, administrative procedures, educational practices, and so on" (Rorty, 1998a, p. 326). If we cannot always hope for broad, societywide enlightenment and emancipation, then "melioration," as John Dewey put it, may be a reasonable goal, so "that the specific conditions which exist at one moment, be they comparatively bad or comparatively good, in any event may be bettered" (Dewey, in Campbell, 1995, p. 261). This may be especially important for public administrators who are employed by people embedded in the society that critical theory finds deficient. Such administrators are not usually in a position to call for radical change, but they often are able to propose incremental changes in policy and operating procedures that can make a useful difference to the public.

Theoretical grounding for this more limited approach to social change may be found in the work of Richard Rorty. Rorty shares the postmodern aversion to foundational, universalist ideas; much of his career as a philosopher has been spent deconstructing philosophical foundationalism. Like his predecessor John Dewey, Rorty espouses a pragmatist philosophy of incremental change that is sometimes attacked by radicals and reformers as supportive of the status quo (Campbell, 1995, pp. 225–265). At the same time, he advocates social change to advance democracy and reduce human suffering and humiliation. In the pragmatist mode of focusing on possible futures instead of social metanarratives from the past, Rorty (1998a, p. 234) discards the critical theorist's concerns about capitalism and oppressed classes, since these concerns depend on "the implicit claim that we can do better than a market economy, that we know of a viable option for complex technologically oriented societies. But at the moment, at least, we know of no such option." In place of radical visions of change, Rorty concentrates on hope for a better future, dreaming the sort of "fantasies" that:

can stand on their own without being twined around some large conceptually graspable object. These are the homely, familiar fantasies shared by the educated and the uneducated, by us middle-class intellectuals in U.S. and European universities and by people living in shantytowns outside Lima. They are concrete fantasies about a future in which everybody can get work from which they derive some satisfaction and for which they are decently paid, and in which they are safe from violence and from humiliation. (p. 232)

Given the apparent absence of general social theory in Rorty's work that could be used to ground action, his commitment to social betterment begs the question of what values underlie his normative choices. Rorty portrays himself as a leftist reformer (1998b), acknowledging that "to say that history is 'the history of class struggle,' is still true, if it is interpreted to mean that in every culture, under every form of government, and in every imaginable situation . . . the people who have already got their hands on money and power will lie, cheat, and steal in order to make sure that they and their descendants monopolize both forever" (Rorty, 1999, p. 206).

John Dewey said much the same thing. Arguing that free access to information is the best way for the general public to control the excesses of economic elites, he wrote in 1927 that "As long as interests of pecuniary profit are powerful, and a public has not located and identified itself, those who have this interest will have an unresisted motive for tampering with the springs of political action in all that affects them" (Dewey, 1927, p. 182).

We have come full circle, back to the broader questioning of social conditions, economics, power, and human behavior we might expect of critical theorists. Rorty's view of social change may not include yearning to scrap the current political economy or implement a single version of utopia, but his desire for betterment comes close to those of leftist sociologist C. Wright Mills, later John Dewey (Tilman, 1984, chap. 8), and Habermas (Rorty, 1989, pp. 65–67). With the critical theorists, each of these people expresses concern about the human condition in advanced Western nations. Frankfurt theorists were forced by circumstances to abandon hope of a revolution of workers, and their vision of broad, societywide emancipation does not seem to fit today's societies. However, these three reformers share with critical theorists a desire for social change that meliorates social conditions they deplore.

Critical Public Administration Scholarship

Without identifying specifically with the ideas of one theorist or school of thought, we agree to some extent with the critical theory analysis of society as a set of material conditions that offer fertile grounds for social change.

We also sympathize with the reformer's view that, given the world in which we live, we should do what we can and be satisfied with incremental or localized action. History is not a unitary fact, but is what we make of it today, and the future is a social construction. This is not to deny the facticity of society as it appears in the present. Rather, "we live not in a settled and finished world, but in one which is going on, and where our main task is prospective, and where retrospect—and all knowledge as distinct from thought is retrospect—is of value in the solidity, security, and fertility it affords our dealings with the future" (Dewey, in Campbell, 1995, p. 61). Rorty (1998, p. 320) notes that, for "a naturalistic historicist" like Dewey, "every form of social life is likely, sooner or later, to freeze over into something the more imaginative and restless spirits of the time will see as 're-pressive' and 'distorting.'" Thus, "as Marx and Foucault helped us see, today's chains are often forged from the hammers that struck off yesterday's. As Foucault was more inclined to admit than Marx, this sequence of hammers into chains *is* unlikely to end with the invention of hammers that cannot be forged into chains—hammers that are purely rational, with no ideological alloy. Still, the chains might, with luck, get a little lighter and easier to break each time" (p. 320).

Given these assumptions about society, action, and history, the question becomes what academicians in public administration can or should do, within their scholarly work, in the service of meaningful change. We work in a field inclined toward the technical and instrumental, during a time when powerful forces breathe new life into the project of separating democratic will formation from administration, reanimating the politics-administration dichotomy that many thought had disappeared. These forces seek to collapse the two realms of thought in public administration, the social/political and the organizational/managerial, into one, the organizational/managerial (Ventriss, 2000). This leads to dominance of mechanistic, descriptive thinking that ignores meaning and purpose, as the last vestiges of traditional public service values and "new public administration" give way to "new public management" and the "technicist episteme" (White & McSwain, 1990) is fully realized. It is not easy for public administration scholars who care about social hope and broader social inquiry to work toward a better future in such an intellectual environment. Rorty (1999, p. 121), following Dewey (and speaking in particular of the American setting), suggests that higher education should help students think of themselves as part of "a tradition of increasing liberty and rising hope," by discussing the history of a nation seeking independence, freeing the slaves, enfranchising women, restraining the robber barons, and so on. In addition to fulfilling a vocational training role, universities should encourage teachers to provoke students into "self-creation" by making "vivid and concrete the failure of the country of which we remain loyal citizens to live up to its own ideals—the failure of America to be what it knows it ought to become" (p. 123). Not everyone will want, or be able, to do this. It may be too controversial to be decided in faculty meetings, and it is not "the sort of thing that can be easily explained to the governmental authorities or the trustees who supply the cash" (p. 123).

This is indeed a hopeful vision of teaching interpretive and sometimes critical history that allows students to comprehend a world more complex, divisive, and difficult than the one in which they have grown up believing. But this vision may strike some as too optimistic, breezing too easily over the history and nature of social institutions and their effects on humans and the physical environment. Marcuse (1964, p. 226) helps pull us back to grapple with these basic issues, doing so with simple stories like this:

> I take a walk in the country. Everything is as it should be: Nature at its best. Birds, sun, soft grass, a view through the trees of the mountains, nobody around, no radio, no smell of gasoline. Then the path turns and ends on the highway. I am back among the billboards, service stations, motels, and roadhouses. I was in a National Park, and I now know that this was not reality. It was a "reservation," something that is being preserved like a species dying out. If it were not for the government, the billboards, hot dog stands, and motels would long since have invaded that piece of Nature. I am grateful to the government; we have it much better than before.

The bittersweet paradox of false consciousness pervades this story. Over time, people become so accustomed to the way things are in a society of capitalist technical rationality that they no longer know that alternatives could exist. History is written to match the values of contemporary society, which is shaped by the economic imperatives of the market. Everything collapses into, as Marcuse said, one dimension, from which there seems to be no escape. The past is a unified march into the only present that could exist and the future must be more of the same. We are grateful for what it offers and would resist the suggestion that we have forfeited much in exchange for little.

"Clio at the Crossroads": Writing Critical History

What would historical methods look like if we were writing critical history? Clio, the muse of history, is at a crossroads.[1] According to Berkhofer (1995, p. 25), the adoption by historians of the linguistic, interpretative, and rhetorical turns has "changed some vocabulary and introduced some new subjects and ways of handling that subject matter" into the discipline of history. However, they "pale beside the challenge to the fundamental presuppositions of traditional historical writing and practice posed by the various turns and contradictory problems in the human sciences" (p. 25). He continues:

> While historicization supposedly solves the problems of theory in other disciplines, these historicizations in turn do not solve the theoretical problems those disciplines pose for doing history in these postmodern, poststructuralist times. Just what forms any historicization can possibly take after the severe challenges literary and rhetorical theorists themselves issued to traditional ways of representing history is the question we need to consider at this moment in the practice of history. The challenges are clear enough; the proper responses are far less certain, despite the enthusiasm for a new cultural history and new historicisms in general. (p. 25)

Although the proper responses are uncertain, there are a few examples in public administration of (re)constructing a past that goes beyond the great story, calling into question, by the nature of the historical narrative, the ideological system or episteme privileged by the dominant narrative. For teachers/scholars who would teach/write nonstandard history in which the present appears as an uneasy resting point rather than a natural result and the future is less than certain, there exists kindred work of critical historical understanding. This work shows it is possible to offer views that provoke, generate new awareness, maybe even enable public practitioners or scholars to rethink their "fantasies" of the future. There is not space in this paper to fully explore such work, but a few examples may be identified (with apologies to other, equally appropriate work not cited).

One recent example, mentioned earlier, is Camilla Stivers's *Bureau Men, Settlement Women: Constructing Public Administration in the Progressive Era* (2000a). In this book, Stivers tells the story of how circumstances affected the formation of knowledge and practice in American public administration as we know it today. She tells the story of the construction of public administration "in a way that calls into question the field's rather taken-for-granted methodological quality and puts it back into its historical context, a framework in which science, business, and gender are equally important and in which its political dimensions are made clear" (p. 2). She offers a critical history of public administration by deconstructing the Progressive-era construction of contemporary public administration, showing how what we select as important and meaningful ideas and practices "brings into sharp relief certain aspects of that society and casts others into shadow"

(p. 3). She continues: "Choices on the part of intellectuals, particularly in social science, about what is important or meaningful in the social dynamics around them set in motions patterns of thought that become important conceptual currency. Circulated in public, these concepts become means by which, for good or ill, people interpret the circumstances of their lives and decide what is possible to do or worth doing" (p. 3).

Other examples of historical interpretation breaking out of the dominant paradigm include another book by Stivers, with Cheryl Simrell King and collaborators. *Government Is Us: Public Administration in an Anti-Government Era* (King & Stivers 1998) includes essays that explore alternative interpretations of American governance history, critically analyzing relationships of political and economic power that were formative of founding-era debates and subsequent events, and linking them to contemporary challenges and visions for the future. In another example, *Legitimacy in Public Administration: A Discourse Analysis* (1997), O.C. McSwite traces the effects of the founding-era victory of the Federalists, representing established wealth and power, over the Anti-Federalists, representing the ordinary citizen. McSwite reconstructs the Anti-Federalist vision of a cooperative society, proposing a "collaborative pragmatism" much like Rorty's updated Deweyan approach. It is a joint problem-solving setting with dialogue free of foundational presuppositions and domination by people who think their way is the only way, and it leads experimentally and incrementally to a better future. Finally, in *Citizen Governance: Leading American Communities into the Twenty-first Century* (1998), Richard Box portrays the history of local public affairs in terms of domination by elite groups. Though the forms and practices have changed since the American colonial era, influence and domination remain and continue to significantly shape and constrain the activities of citizens and public administrators.

Similar attention to unpacking the historical assumptions of the dominant contemporary culture can be found in related fields. Robert Zinn's *A People's History of the United States* (1999) is written from the point of view of those who have been politically and economically marginalized and exploited and, typically, are missing from most histories. A PBS "miniseries" of this work is currently in production, indicating the recognition of the importance of critical historical analysis in popular culture. Historian Gordon Wood exhaustively documents relations between common people and those with wealth and power in the founding era in the book *The Creation of the American Republic, 1776–1787* (1969), portraying politics in the era as a struggle between these groups. In *Democracy and Capitalism: Property, Community, and the Contradictions of Modern Social*

Thought (1986), economists Samuel Bowles and Herbert Gintis suggest that American history may be understood as a series of accommodations between the wealthy and everyone else. These accommodations allowed sufficient personal liberty to keep popular uprising to a minimum. Bowles and Gintis argue that the United States was able for some time to escape the tension between personal rights and capitalist accumulation of property experienced in Europe because it had abundant land available for settlement. Taught history often confines the idea of social conflict to large-scale international events such as world wars, but in *Civic Wars: Democracy and Public Life in the American City during the Nineteenth Century* (1997), historian Mary Ryan captures the tumultuous character of life in nineteenth-century urban America. She examines conflict in New York, New Orleans, and San Francisco over issues of race, nationality, religion, gender, and wealth, conflict that frequently included disorder and mob violence. Ryan (1997, p. 7) writes: "Democratic politics and decisions about the conjoined life of a polity are worked out in an unremitting practice whereby citizens name, assert, and give meaning to themselves and one another." This is not a process of inevitable progress or the triumph of technical rationality, as Ryan notes in summarizing her findings from the three cities: "On the simplest level this history warns against looking to the past for some harmonious, decorous, unified public sphere that will serve as the singular model of democratic politics. Conversely, it begs attention and appreciation for the shrill-voiced, loud-mouthed, rowdy, demanding, contentious citizenry. Democracy is a politics not of unity but of opposition" (p. 311).

At the level of the organization, two examples may serve to illustrate critical historical analysis of the connection between social conditions and conditions in the workplace. One is *Organizational America* (1979), by William Scott and David Hart, which describes the transition, from the nineteenth century into the twentieth, from the "individual imperative" to the "organizational imperative." As the result of this change, people are controlled by modern organizations using *"universal behavioral techniques to integrate individuals and groups into mutually reinforcing relationships with advancing technology in order to achieve system goals efficiently"* [italics in original] (p. 4). The behavioral techniques are drawn from behavioral science and are *"used to obtain obedience to managerial instructions"* [italics in original] (p. 4).

Roy Jacques explores this individual-organization transition in relation to the social and personal impacts of employment. In the book *Manufacturing the Employee: Management Knowledge from the Nineteenth to Twenty-first Centuries* (1996), he sets out to "create a more comprehensive forum for discussing the problems of tomorrow by articulating ways that today's problems are constrained by yesterday's" (p. ix). Until the late nineteenth century, most people worked for themselves on farms or in shops and work and personal life were integrated within a community. With the coming of modern organizations, work was separated from home, family, and community, with significant effects on individual autonomy, family and gender relations, and the content of work.

Some of the authors discussed in these examples would identify their theoretical approach as critical theory, others not, but all share a commitment to interpreting history with a probing, critical mindset that goes beyond the standard presentations of the dominant culture. For them, a dialogical past has brought us to a present that is part of a process, rather than a reasoned and static result. Each author believes such critical historical interpretation to be essential for hopeful construction of the future.

We take our orders from this belief—that it is not possible to "rewrite the present" without engaging in critical historical interpretation. As we have outlined in this final section, there are some examples of critical historical interpretation in public administration and in other fields, including the field of history. We urge public administrator practitioners and scholars to take our charge to engage in critical historical interpretation seriously— to commit what Marcuse (1964) called the "great refusal," refusing, at least in some times and places, to let one's work continue to play a systems-affirming role. Without this kind of practice and scholarship, however difficult it may be, it is impossible to "rewrite the present"—all that is possible is to marginally revise the texts already written for us.

Note

1. The expression "Clio at the crossroads" is from Berkhofer, 1995, p. 25.

— 4 —

Critical Theory and the Paradox of Discourse

The work of public administration theorists who argue for a broader sphere of administrative discretion falls into three broad paradigms: the legitimacy paradigm, the guardian paradigm, and the critical paradigm. Legitimacy theorists argue for recognition within the Constitutional framework, and guardian theorists argue for more discretion for administrators to govern for the uninformed public. Neither view has much practical impact because neither fits American attitudes toward government. The critical paradigm advocates providing citizens with information so they may take action and free themselves from domination by elites. This critical view involves less, rather than more, formal power for professional administrators and puts them at odds with the elected officials who employ them. The paper seeks to determine whether this view of the role of the public administrator accurately portrays the nature of the relationship between citizens and government and whether the public administrator can be an effective agent of change by becoming an information provider instead of seeking greater institutional power.

Much of the literature of public administration theory is concerned with determining how much discretion public professionals should exercise and whom they should serve. The neutrality model of administrative discretion

From *American Review of Public Administration*, vol. 25, no. 1 (March 1995): 1–19.
Copyright © 1995 Sage Publications, Inc. Reprinted with permission.

calls for the public administrator to accept whatever conditions exist and carry out directives from those in power. Though this instrumental view of the administrative role avoids problems raised by the politics-administration question, the attention of academicians and many practitioners is focused on altering existing relationships between the political and administrative spheres.

The legitimacy model is a prevalent normative view in this area; it seeks institutional legitimacy for public administration and greater discretion for professional public administrators. The critical theory model seeks to alter the political-administrative relationship not by attaining greater recognition and discretion, but by minimizing professional control and transferring knowledge and decision-making capability from government to citizens.

A normative view of the role of the public professional that has useful and concrete impact in the daily work world cannot be built only upon the value preferences of theorists; rather, it must be built upon a recognition of values, desired end results, and a pragmatic understanding of the cultural, economic, and political context within which American public administration occurs. Though theoretical work within the legitimacy model leads to greater understanding of institutional relationships, it has little practical relevance for public administrators because societal trends and deeply held American beliefs run counter to the desire to achieve greater autonomy for public professionals. It is easy enough to advocate a normative position, suggesting the best role for public administrators, but arriving at a position that can have real effect requires taking the context of administration into account. This context renders the legitimacy model ineffective in dealing with contemporary problems facing practicing professionals.

Given the limited usefulness of the legitimacy model in shaping public administrative practice, we turn our attention to the critical theory model. This model downplays claims for superior decision making by public professionals in relation to the public, instead emphasizing the role of the professional in allowing citizens to express their own vision of the future. Key premises of the critical theory model as applied to public administration are that political structures allow for control by elites and that open exchange between citizens and between public administrators and citizens can change these structures by redistributing knowledge and the ability to use it in public policy making. This discussion, or "discourse," shifts the locus of policy initiation and decision making from the professional administrator to the citizen.

The sections below examine these features of the critical theory model and evaluate how it affects the public administrator's role. The conclusion claims that interaction between administrators and citizens can be a powerful tool for opening political systems to greater public self-determination. Paradoxically, the effectiveness of the public professional administrator can be increased by relinquishing claims to legitimacy and working with, instead of against, values that favor citizens rather than professional control.

Values Underlying the Models

The Legitimacy Model

Writers desiring increased legitimacy for public administration usually focus on the national level of government. The question of legitimacy centers on the relationship of public administration to the Constitution and the nature of the founding period (Rohr, 1986, 1993; Spicer & Terry, 1993; Stivers, 1993; Wamsley et al., 1987). Though there is confusion about what "legitimacy" means (Warren, 1993, pp. 250–252), a legitimized public administration would seem to be one the public respects, that has more authority and discretion to act independently than at present, and that is given the status of a somewhat equal partner to the existing branches of government.

Legitimacy may be seen as necessary because the complex nature of modern society often causes a muddled and ineffective political leadership. Also, the public may have lost the capacity to carry out its responsibilities because of ignorance or indifference. The expertise of public professionals can steer government out of this morass, and, carried to its logical extreme, the search for legitimacy might culminate in a guardian class of administrators who make decisions they believe citizens choose not to make or cannot make competently (Fox & Cochran, 1990).

The idea of increased administrative legitimacy may be criticized for lacking justification within the American political tradition, for being irrelevant given the existing dominance of the administrative state, or for advocating an antidemocratic administrative elite. Greater legitimacy for public administration could be a path toward a more democratic, equalitarian, and humane society. Alternatively, it could lead to diminution of personal freedom as "domination functions as administration, and in the overdeveloped areas of mass consumption, the administered life becomes the good life of the whole" (Marcuse, 1964, p. 255), resulting in "the Happy Consciousness—the belief that the real is rational and that the system delivers the goods" (p. 84).

These questions about the legitimacy model are important, but they lack clear answers and reach far into the future. A more immediate and telling critique is that of pragmatism. No one would deny that administrative theorists should explore the fundamental nature of contemporary society and its relationship to public administration. However, theorizing about legitimacy occupies a significant part of the effort of theory building in public administration, so it makes sense to assess the likely impact such an investment in time and energy may have on the actual practice of administration.

The short-run effect of legitimacy advocacy on the practice of public administration is negligible. Declarations of the desirability of institutional legitimacy or greater discretionary authority for public administrators may soothe people irritated with what they perceive as the unfortunate effects of bureaucrat bashing or conservative ideology. However, such declarations do not change the nature of the culture that surrounds administration, nor do they reach into the places where most of the work of American public administration takes place. There may be some administrators in large organizations who have the time to consider such questions, the opportunity to take action based on the legitimacy model, and the ability to "hide" their activities from political accountability. But these administrative advantages, if that is what they are, are available to administrators in smaller agencies, especially local agencies, in limited quantities.

The long-term impact of the legitimacy model may not be substantial either. Considering an institutional change that can become real only by fundamentally changing the underlying values and legal structure of society serves a purpose in identifying the need for changes in the existing situation. However, given pressing problems of public governance, it may be unproductive to spend too much time on ideas that have little chance of influencing the course of affairs. An honest appraisal of the possibility of implementing increased authority and discretion for professional public administrators, aside from the question of the size of government generally, must conclude that the vast majority of the American people simply will not have it. It is not necessary to characterize the time in which we live as one of great skepticism about government to reach this conclusion. At any time, Americans, faced with the idea of a powerful and independent administrative class, would ask questions like: What would change if we had it? Would public administrators have power and wealth instead of private-sector entrepreneurs? Would they create a "leveler" society, distributing resources equally, and what would this do to economic life? Why should we expect these people to do any "better" than our politicians, or for that matter the bureaucrats of totalitarian states? Why should I give away whatever ability I have to decide the fate of my nation, state, or community to a clique of nonaccountable technicians?

This pragmatic critique is not intended to lock discussion of public administration into an instrumental, status-quo vision in theory or practice. Rather, the intent is to identify ideas that we could reasonably expect to have an impact in the foreseeable future, and it does not appear that the legitimacy model is such an idea.

The Critical Theory Model

The critical theory model has for some time occupied a marginal position in public administration theory. Denhardt (1981a) called for increased application of critical theory in public administration. White (1986) discussed critical theory as an alternative to traditional positivistic research, and several authors have used variations of critical theory in their work. Nevertheless, critical theory has remained peripheral to the larger body of work in public administration theory.

With "its roots in Hegelian philosophy, specifically Hegel's view of history as the unfolding of reason and the freedom which reason implies" (Denhardt, 1981a, pp. 629), critical theory seeks to "reveal society for what it is, to unmask its essence and mode of operation and to lay the foundations for human emancipation through deep-seated social change" (Burrell & Morgan, 1979, p. 284). What critical theorists think society is has emerged with modern urban-industrial society, which is administered by huge Weberian public and private bureaucracies. This society is built upon the market model of the citizen as individual utility-maximizer within a technological, consumerist system (Macpherson, 1977, pp. 77–82).

Development of this system has been facilitated by the use of science and technology, "purposive-rational" ways of dealing with issues of social, economic, and political life. This purposive rationality "extends to the correct choice among strategies, the appropriate application of technologies, and the efficient establishment of systems" (Habermas, 1970, p. 82), crowding out individual consideration of life options and replacing it with a "one-dimensional" ideology in which "the political needs of society become individual needs and aspirations, their satisfaction promotes business and the commonwealth, and the whole appears to be the very embodiment of Reason" (Marcuse, 1964, p. ix).

The problem with this situation, according to critical theorists, is that, "by virtue of its structure, purposive-rational action is the exercise of control" (Habermas, 1970, p. 82), in itself a form of domination. Because the ideology of mass production, consumption, and the good life of material security becomes universal, people are unable to evaluate critically their circumstances and consider alternative ways of living. Though they strive to conform and achieve, they are left with a "vague malaise, free-floating dissatisfaction, irrational behavior patterns, etc.—in short, a situation of frustration and unhappiness which is not recognized for what it is" (Geuss, 1981, p. 81).

This trap of superficial happiness and deep-seated malaise that does not reach conscious awareness is a state of delusion called "false consciousness." As a remedy, critical theory advocates political action in which people are freed from their false consciousness by giving them the knowledge they need to make their own choices. The desired "final state is one in which the agents are free of false consciousness—they have been enlightened . . . [and] they have been emancipated" (Geuss, 1981, p. 58). People resist being emancipated because knowledge of their condition threatens their feeling of security and many do not believe they are kept in a position of material satisfaction and psychological dissatisfaction by an economic elite. For the critical theorist, the majority is:

> constantly bombarded with intensive advertising propaganda to show how well off they are and how fortunate they are to have all the things they have. They are trained to accent accelerating consumption as the inevitable way of their lives. And they are admonished at all times not to mess around with the horn of plenty because such actions will obliterate their jobs and their consumption potential. This is not a context from which militant masses, bent upon reform, are likely to arise. (Scott & Hart, 1979, p. 219)

The critical theory model, unlike much of the writing in public administration theory, explicitly recognizes the political constraints inherent in the ecology of public administration practice. In the society of the critical theorist, the administrator is employed by those who hold, or who represent those who hold, power gained through control of the market. Though the partially democratic nature of the capitalist political system allows public access to policy, the reality of elite control based on power and wealth cannot be avoided. Because the public is not aware of purposive-rational domination, it cannot effectively participate in public governance nor step outside its condition to evaluate the need for change.

In contrast to the legitimacy model, in which professional public administrators become the focus of meaningful change (such as redistributing societal wealth with the goal of "social equity"), critical theory aims to create conditions in which a fully conscious public enacts change. In these conditions, public administrators do not strive for greater power, autonomy, and recognition. Instead, they give away knowledge and the power to make decisions to the people who are affected by those decisions. Paradoxically, this giving away is assumed to bring the administrator much closer to desired policy outcomes than would be possible by increasing professional control.

Such an action is risky for the administrator in two ways: The professional may be disciplined or fired for stirring up political currents politicians dislike, and the public, once emancipated, may choose policies not to the administrator's liking. The visions of a better future public administrators hold are not monolithic, nor are those of the general public, whether it is deluded or emancipated. For critical theorists or administrators to advocate a particular view of the future is contrary to emancipation's intent, which is to allow people to make their own choices when fully informed of the alternatives available to them. In so doing, as Terry Cooper (1991, p. 167) put it, the public administrator "is responsible for upholding the sovereignty of the people while also making available to them certain technical skills and knowledge."

The introductory section above introduced two premises of the critical theory model that we should examine in assessing the usefulness of the model to public administration. The first is that political structures allow for control by elites, the second that discourse between citizens and between public administrators and citizens can change these structures by redistributing knowledge and the ability to use it in public policy making. The next section explores the nature of elite control, using the local community as the unit of analysis.

The Relationship Between the Powerful and the Governed

The Literature of Community Power

There is no lack of research in the area of national or subnational power structures (see Ricci, 1971; Waste, 1986). The field of public administration tends to discuss the administrator's role without an explicit assessment of the nature of the political setting that constrains administrative action. This tendency ignores the importance for public administration of what, at the local level, Waste (1989) called "the ecology of city policymaking." Because much of the day-to-day interaction between citizens and administrators occurs at the local level, it makes sense to start there to find whether the critical paradigm is correct in assuming that an elite group controls the public policy agenda.

The literature of community power structures contains several notable milestones such as the Lynds' studies of Muncie, Indiana, in the 1920s and 1930s (1937), Floyd Hunter's (1953) work in Atlanta in the early 1950s, and Robert Dahl's (1961) study of New Haven in the late 1950s. In the post–World War II period and into the 1970s there was a contentious debate between "elite" theorists and "pluralist" theorists that became deadlocked and fruitless. Elite theorists used theoretical constructs and research methodologies that resulted in findings supporting the critical view of control of communities by small, closed, cohesive groups. Using different techniques, pluralists also found governance by small groups, but the groups were open and accessible to the public and had changing membership depending on issues (like urban renewal, public school governance, etc.) (Waste, 1986, pp. 13–25).

Beginning in the 1970s, a variety of approaches offered alternative ways to examine community power. Harrigan (1989, p. 191) grouped these approaches into five areas: neo-Marxist and structural; Harvey Molotch's growth machine theory; Peterson's unitary interest theory; Stone's systematic power and regime theories; and the pluralist counterattack. Each of these ways of looking at community power contains ideas useful to practicing public administrators.

While the elite and pluralist writers debated the form of community power structures, research continued in the field of community governance and leadership styles, as evidenced by works such as Banfield and Wilson's *City Politics* (1963), Kotter and Lawrence's *Mayors in Action* (1974), Loveridge's *City Managers in Legislative Politics* (1971), and Williams and Adrian's *Four Cities* (1963). After some years as a local government practitioner, studying the literature of community power as an academician, and teaching these concepts to midcareer practitioners, I have found that a handful of models are especially powerful in describing everyday reality and in helping practitioners to understand their working environment. One of these, "growth machine" theory, grew out of the elite-pluralist debate in the field of urban politics. Another, the "four cities" model of Williams and Adrian, came from research into community governance in the early 1960s and presents four community orientations to the relationship of citizens and community leaders.

The Growth Machine

Much of the early writing about community power and governance described phenomena without adequately explaining their underlying causes. The growth machine model Molotch proposed in 1976 hypothesized that local politics is driven by the desire of those owning or controlling land and buildings to make a profit. This elite, called the "growth machine," is composed of landowners, speculators, builders, and the professional and business classes that profit from their activities (lawyers, bankers, newspaper publishers, etc.). They control the public policy agenda through non–decision making (keeping important questions from arising), making decisions in a dull round of meetings about special districts, financing, and others, and diverting public attention from their activities by creating a "we-feeling" of community, using athletic teams and community events to instill "a spirit of civic jingoism regarding the 'progress' of the locality" (Molotch, 1976, p. 315). As a result, "the city is, for those who count, a growth machine" (p. 310).

Other theorists have recognized the primacy of land use in the local political economy (e.g., Peterson, 1981), but Molotch's model combines an awareness of market forces, land use as the central feature of the local economy, and the elite's use of diversionary rhetoric and activities to convince the general public that their vision of the future of the community is good for everybody. Several researchers have done directly related empirical work since the introduction of the growth machine model. Among other findings, the growth machine appears to have some validity in explaining mayoral attitudes toward growth (Maurer & Christenson, 1982), and the public may well be at odds with its growth-oriented elected representatives (Anglin, 1990). The strength of the growth machine can vary significantly from community to community, and some resist it actively (Logan & Molotch, 1987, pp. 209–228). But it takes energy to resist the basic market forces of profiting from land use, and in the majority of places, over time the political process is driven by "people dreaming, planning, and organizing themselves to make money from property" (p. 12).

To the extent the growth machine model reflects reality in a given community, it will be difficult for administrators to serve as a vehicle for citizen emancipation and at the same time keep their job. The elite have a significant financial interest in keeping the public ignorant and uninvolved. A professional who attempts to inform people who may not agree with the growth machine's goals incurs considerable risk; risk that may produce a rewarding result but that may also create conflict, personal insecurity, and professional uncertainty. In short, if the elite attack a professional for stirring up resistance to the growth machine, how far should the professional push this course of action? How much risk should professionals assume, and how can they be certain that serving a perceived broader public interest is more "right" than serving the governing elite?

"Four Cities"

The growth machine is a compelling explanatory tool for local government practitioners who have dealt with issues of planning and development. A major weakness of the model is that, in making the point that land use drives the local political economy, it slights consideration of the differences between communities. Williams and Adrian's research (1963), described in their book, *Four Cities,* explicitly identified several such differences. Though it may be argued that the growth machine dynamic is present in each of the four community types Williams and Adrian describe, these communities nevertheless exhibited different approaches to the role of community governance in citizen lives. Williams and Adrian (1963) described the four city types as follows:

1. *Promoting economic growth.* "The object of government is to see that the community grows in population and/or total wealth" (p. 23).
2. *Providing and securing life's amenities.* The central purpose of government is to create a "quiet and peaceful environment for the home" (p. 25).
3. *Maintaining traditional services ("caretaker" government).* "Private decisions regarding the allocation of personal resources are lauded over governmental allocation through taxation," and, "The caretaker image is associated with a policy of opposition to zoning, planning, and other regulations of the use of real property" (p. 27).
4. *Arbitrating among conflicting interests.* "Emphasis is placed upon the process rather than the substance of governmental action" in the pluralistic arbiter community (p. 28).

This typology has been criticized as partially failing to identify "substantive objectives the community can maximize" (Peterson, 1981, p. 31), but it presents a range of community characteristics found in few other conceptualizations of the nature of communities. Like any model, it could be improved, and it describes many, but not all, situations that may be encountered in the real world. Nevertheless, the descriptions of community types in the model make sense in relation to common knowledge about urban places. The community that promotes economic growth is a common type and matches Molotch's growth machine city. The exclusive suburban enclave that emphasizes life's amenities is also well known, as is the diverse, conflictual arbiter city in which many groups, coalitions, and individuals compete for political advantage. The caretaker city may seem somewhat unfamiliar, although I live in such a city, a place where government is mistrusted and is expected to be as limited in scope as possible.

Diversity in Community Orientation

The importance of the four cities model to the question of elite control is that we can expect the motivations of key political actors and the ways in which they organize to achieve their objectives to be different in different places. Because of this variation, administrators wishing to enlighten and emancipate the public act contingent upon the specifics of the community setting.

Not every community requires administrative intervention to correct a knowledge imbalance between the governing group and citizens. Some places have open and accessible governing processes; others are relatively closed and exclusive. In any case, the goals of governing groups cannot always be determined from the presence of open or closed governance. For example, Molotch's growth machine can exist with or without the manipulative activities he portrays. It is not unreasonable to envision a community in which there is informed and enthusiastic consensus about the desirability of growth. In other communities there may be open conflict over growth, with the growth machine faction "winning" politically much of the time (Vogel & Swanson, 1989). In such places, control of information is not the problem; the source of the conflict is fundamental disagreement about ends. There are also communities in which resistance to unfettered growth is a dominant and lasting feature of the political system (Lewis, 1991). Finally, issues other than growth may be of primary importance in a community despite the market imperative for making profits from land.

The human inclination to dominate others for personal gain is timeless; a Lockean concern for allowing liberty while limiting the negative effects of this inclination was at the center of the constitutional debates (McDonald, 1985). However, the discussion above leads to the conclusion that political activity can be based on a variety of motivations and that the level of citizen awareness and involvement is variable as well. I have observed five local governments in depth as a practitioner and have seen a range of governmental concerns and citizen awareness. A quick summary of the nature of the governance systems in these five places can serve as an anecdotal illustration of the variety to be found in communities:

Place No. 1. This was the type of community Molotch described, with a strong pro-growth orientation, a small, relatively unchanging governing elite of businesspeople, and a largely uninformed citizenry.

Place No. 2. This was a rural area with few incorporated cities, residents who wanted to be as free from government as possible, and not much attention being directed toward growth. The primary concern of the active and involved citizenry was limiting the role of government in their lives.

Place No. 3. Growth was the central concern in this community, with an emerging opposition to the pro-growth orientation of the downtown business group that had always controlled the city's politics. (The city was later to become a center for pro-environment, managed-growth sentiment with much citizen involvement.)

Place No. 4. Growth was also the central concern in this community, with open conflict and heated debate. The governing group was open to new membership, and the public agenda was characterized by intense citizen involvement and widespread knowledge of the technical and substantive issues surrounding physical and economic growth.

Place No. 5. Growth ranked low in priority as a concern in this town, and keeping taxes low ranked high. The governing system was open to everyone, though few participated, and large landowners blocked governmental actions that threatened their ability to make profit from development. Citizen awareness of issues was relatively poor, characterized by apathy and lack of information.

In Williams and Adrian's typology, Place 1 was concerned with economic development, and Places 3 and 4 were experiencing a clash between the economic development focus and the orientation toward securing life's amenities. Places 2 and 5 were caretaker communities concerned with maintaining traditional services at low cost.

Of the five communities described above, Places 1 and 3 were ripe for the sort of discourse the critical theory model advocates. The interests of individuals and groups in Place 5 were poorly articulated and had not taken shape around specific issues other than low taxes, so there was little room for discourse except that relating to technical matters of management. In Places 2 and 4, the level of citizen awareness and involvement was intense. Professional aid in these places would be oriented toward injecting professional rationality into a politicized discourse.

Though small and unsystematic, this sample of local communities supports the conclusion that generalization is difficult. Not every place is controlled by an elite, with citizens in need of emancipation through discourse. Of those that are, the specific needs vary. Finding that the nature of community governance and the need for professional facilitation of discourse varies does not mean the critical theory model is inaccurate or lacking in usefulness, but that its application is contingent on time, place, and local conditions. Where the conditions are right for application of the model, how effective can it be?

Discourse Effectiveness

Discourse Legitimacy

Americans tend to believe they have a right to participate in the democratic process when and where they wish. Many people may be disenchanted with politics, many may feel powerless, and some may point out that the founders of the nation were antidemocratic elitists who never intended the masses to be equal partners in governance (Dye & Ziegler, 1987; Stivers, 1993). However, after two centuries of evolution of American political and constitutional tradition, the expectation of free access is prevalent, whether or not it is reality (Schattschneider, 1960, pp. 126–139).

The value placed on free access to democratic decision making is evidence of the implicit understanding that knowledge and political control are directly related. In a modern information-based society, virtually everyone is aware of the impact of information and the way it is used to influence governmental outcomes. To the extent that elites—national, state, or local—can control the agenda and content of the public debate over important issues, they can control results. But the spread of knowledge breaks down control relationships in "the twilight of hierarchy" (Cleveland, 1985) so that the power of information and of making it openly available is considerable.

When public administrators uncouple their behaviors from the interests of governing elites and serve all involved citizens equally in revealing the substantive rationality of alternative visions of the future (White, 1990, pp. 132–150), citizens have the tools to create the change they want, whatever it may be. Such administrative behavior may not be explicitly constitutionally "legitimate." However, it is legitimate to the extent that it is not proscribed by the people's representatives. That is, elected representatives (Congress, state legislatures, city councils, county boards of commissioners, governing boards of special districts) have the legitimate authority to stop the efforts of administrators to enable free discourse. They may do so by order and ultimately by discharging the offending administrator. If they do not do so, the administrator's actions are by definition legitimate in that they are sanctioned by those with the relevant constitutional or legal authority.

Involvement in Discourse

Often we think of administrators involved in discourse with the public as being those at the top of organizational hierarchies, those who interact with citizen policy makers to shape the content of public policy. Public organizations contain a variety of boundary-spanning positions in which public employees interact frequently or constantly with the public, but not all of these positions are involved in discourse that communicates information that could alter policies. Examples would include a motor vehicles clerk or welfare department intake worker, positions in which communication with the public is routine, limited in scope, and only infrequently causes change beyond the immediate worksite.

However, many middle- and lower-level administrators have meaningful discourse with the public. Examples would include a planner or engineer who works with citizen advisory committees or a police community affairs officer who works to improve relations between police and citizens. Such people have the opportunity to communicate their agency's mission and vision of the future to citizens. They also have the opportunity to interject professional knowledge and opinions that may not correspond to the agency view, information that may allow citizens greater understanding and opportunity for action that changes the agency-citizen relationship. By definition, then, the question of discourse relates to those administrators high enough in the hierarchy to be at or near the politics-administration interface and also to those whose boundary-spanning jobs take them beyond the language of technical interchange with the public into discussion of alternative policies.

In addition to public administrators who are involved in discourse with the public, many are not directly involved with citizens but contribute significantly to constructive change in public administration. Though critical theory focuses on discourse as a means of altering the distribution of political power, there are other ways to contribute to the pool of knowledge available to professional and citizen decision makers and to increase the rationality of decisions. In concentrating on discourse with citizens as an instrument of social change, we narrow the pool of affected public administrators, but administrators may bring about meaningful change while working in positions that do not include public contact.

The critical theory model envisions discourse as a technique of opening the public agenda to a broad group of citizens to counter governing elites' self-interested control. However, governing bodies may reflect diverse and broadly representative views rather than those of a monolithic elite so that the professional offers the benefits of full and free discussion to the governing body in addition to the general public. In the example given below, discourse with citizens gradually produced a more representative policy-making process, and in some places (like the "arbiter" city described previously) the public agenda may be characterized by open debate. The professional role as facilitator of discourse is different in arbiter cities than in the elite-dominated community, but the value of rational professionalism remains considerable because a public dialogue based solely on the struggle for power can lapse easily enough into factional dominance. Professional provision of information and creation of open discourse remain valuable across a variety of political settings, not all of which fit the model of citizen action to counter control by a unified political elite.

Outcomes of Administrator-Citizen Interaction

Citizen involvement has been used for some time as a tool to alter jurisdictional political agendas. Allowing citizens to influence the operation of programs despite the wishes of local-government officials was a large part of national government initiatives of the 1960s and 1970s (Ross, Levine, & Stedman, 1991, pp. 163–193) and is a common technique in local planning. The orientation toward use of citizen participation for social change has been clearly apparent within professions such as planning (Forester, 1980). Howe and Kaufman (1979) found that urban planners were willing to circumvent established lines of authority to achieve goals they believed to be valid even if their superiors did not. Many planners surveyed believed it acceptable to help citizen groups to overturn official actions their jurisdictions took (Howe & Kaufman, 1979).

Though public administrators often make use of citizen involvement to offset the political advantage the establishment enjoys, it is not necessarily an institutionally accepted mode of professional behavior. For enlightenment and emancipation to function as a guiding philosophy for public administration, it must become engrained in the norms of professional practice, recognized by professionals and the public they serve as a normal, everyday part of how public agencies are run. The question of whether this is a good idea becomes moot if discourse is ineffective in altering policy outcomes.

In the spirit of recognizing the value of "stories managers tell" (Hummel, 1991), an example drawn from one of the five places outlined above may serve to illustrate the usefulness of discourse. Many practitioners have had similar experiences; this set of events is offered only because I can speak about it with some degree of authority in relation to the subject of this paper. In Place 1, I served as a planner tasked with creating a comprehensive land-use plan. The community's governing body and business community had a strong pro-growth orientation and were accustomed to controlling the public policy agenda without serious challenge. This governing group was relatively small, had a consistent membership over time, and was effective in directing community affairs in ways that benefited its members.

As part of the planning, a citizen's committee, required by state law, was formed to help prepare the draft plan. The committee was representative of a broad socioeconomic and geographic cross section of the community. When its members examined issues of type, timing, and location of development, they leaned toward a balance between environmental sensitivity and a sound economy, as contrasted with the high-growth orientation of the governing group. The governing group's reaction to this challenge was to stop the planning process, have an attorney who was a member of the chamber of commerce present the views of the chamber in a public meeting, and direct the citizen's committee to alter its recommendations based on what had been presented.

As the staff person responsible for offering the committee full access to the information needed to make informed (but politically unacceptable) decisions, I was seen as a somewhat misguided troublemaker who should be watched more closely for signs of deviance from the dominant values of the governing group. It was made clear, if indirectly, that my continued employment would depend on a softening of the citizen group's recommendations. This placed me in the situation of persuading citizen committee members to alter their recommendations, which were based on their interpretation of factual information tempered by their value preferences, to fit the financial interests of a small group of business people. This was difficult for some committee members to accept because the committee was a fair representation of the interests of the general public and members had a hard time understanding why a handful of people should override their work.

The final product of this clash of interests was a plan that pleased neither side completely. Despite this, the plan revealed, in easily accessible format, the information needed for informed decisions, something that had occurred in only a fragmentary way before, and the policies adopted moved the community toward greater attention to the environment as opposed to market values. Maybe most important, the citizen's committee became the nucleus of a new group of involved citizens who held broader views of the public interest and good of the community than was typical of some community leaders. The sphere of those involved in policy making was expanded, and citizen involvement, though still regarded with some concern and skepticism, came to be more accepted as part of policy making.

In this case, the model of citizen emancipation through discourse held substantial power. The governing elite felt threatened, and the long-term impacts included greater citizen awareness and governing structures incorporating a wider variety of community opinion. It is difficult to assess the increment of difference between enacted policies following this episode and what would have occurred if citizens had not been given the opportunity for discourse; it probably was measurable but not extremely large. However, it may be just as important to measure the beneficial effects of free discourse in how citizens see themselves and their relationship to their communities as it is to measure them in concrete policy changes.

A public administrator's risk in helping to create a democratically determined agenda of public debate is substantial, as is the courage required to do the work. At the local level, the power of elite groups such as growth machines to stop open consideration of alternative futures is considerable. Use of the critical theory model of discourse is a noble course of action for the public administrator but also involves two types of danger. One type is the danger to the administrator's career if the agency's leaders become so concerned with the administrator's actions that they take disciplinary action. The other type of danger comes from the unpredictability of the outcome of a process of discourse in which the administrator serves as professional information provider rather than as manipulator of discourse to fit a predetermined substantive goal. Citizens who have been enabled by open communication to understand and act on their situation may not share the professional's value preferences. They may instead work toward goals that strike the professional as normatively incorrect, or they may exceed the bounds of their authority and mission as involved citizens. The greater the power of discourse, the greater the risks become.

Conditions Conducive to Discourse

An administrator who acts according to the critical theory model of enlightenment and emancipation accepts the unpredictability of outcomes, convinced that the value of citizen self-determination is greater than that of any particular substantive policy objective. This is not the same thing as the public choice model that defines the public interest as the aggregate of individual interests. The public choice model requires only that citizens measure their self-interests against public policies and pick the proposal that offers the greatest advantage or the least harm to that interest. In the critical theory model, citizens may use self-interest as a decision-making tool, but they must also interact with other citizens and representatives of the public agency, learn and evaluate information relevant to the decision, and consider the impact on others as well as themselves. In such a setting, the substance of individual interests is likely to change so that the decision guide citizens use, rather than isolated self-centered advantage, becomes an informed self-interest in which citizens take into account the larger community as part of their self-interest. This does not require citizens to abandon a sense of individualism or a critical perspective on government's role in society, but rather to be more rational in determining the desired relationship between the individual and the collective community.

Enlightenment and emancipation require free and open discourse. For free and open discourse to occur between citizens and between citizens and public administrators, it is not necessary to have an "ideal" situation (like that envisioned by Habermas) that "assumes a certain kind of symmetry and reciprocity. The symmetry is associated with an equal chance both to initiate communication and to make assertions, while the reciprocity refers to an equal opportunity to make wishes and feelings known, and to provide an assurance that the chances will be equally distributed" (Rasmussen, 1990, p. 64).

In such an ideal setting, people are able to set aside the political, economic, and social conditions that mark the differences between them in their everyday lives and communicate on a level playing field where each person's claims to truth are equally valued. However, in the typical setting of discourse about public issues, the participants bring with them individual characteristics and interest agendas that not only cannot be set aside, but that are in fact the reasons they have gathered together. Also, a legal-institutional context binds the actions of administrators and citizens; they do not conduct discourse in a vacuum, but within a formal framework of laws, programs, finance, and the interests and wishes of the elected governing body of the jurisdiction.

To have a free and open discourse in the typical public setting means that the public administrator must help to create an atmosphere of trust, not only in a general emotional sense, but as an expectation by participating citizens that they will be treated as meaningful actors rather than as disturbing irritants to be calmed, co-opted, led to agree with a predetermined agency agenda. The public professional who accomplishes this sees participative democracy as a core value of professional practice, not as "a cost of doing business rather than the nature and end of governance" (Adams et al., 1990, p. 232).

This means that the administrator must abandon the urge to use "mystery and mastery" (Schon, 1983, pp. 226–230) to control discourse through organizational authority or professional language, instead letting go a considerable degree of control while making possible full public consideration of available and relevant information. As Fox (1992, p. 13) put it, professionals avoid "use of specialized technical knowledge for purposes of obfuscation and exclusion of the noncognoscente." Instead, they move toward making public the dilemma of the professional role in being caught between the imperatives of the organization and the desire to build a constructive relationship with citizens (Schon, 1983, p. 233). In so doing, they describe the interests, agendas, and constraints surrounding the discourse setting as honestly as possible, make clear the boundaries of potential action within the law, provide essential technical information including action alternatives, encourage citizens to decide for themselves how to proceed within the identified constraints, and offer to participate freely in the discussion.

Conclusion: The Practical Application of Critical Theory

This vision of a free and open public discourse is not generalizable to the entire public service in all circumstances. Community opportunities for discourse vary. Also, by definition, this paper explores the role of the administrator who is in a position to carry on meaningful discourse with citizens (or with other professionals) and who wishes to use this position to make change possible through enlightenment and emancipation. The complexity of American government at all levels and the variety of functions within them make it difficult to generalize even within this closely defined population of administrators as potential change agents.

The discussion in this paper supports the critical theory premises that political systems are often dominated by elites and that discourse can lead to constructive change. The view of the public professional presented here is paradoxical, characterized by risk and courage, yet potentially rewarding. Professionals gain legitimacy and authority by giving it away, become part of discourse by maintaining a professional role identity within it, and serve as instruments of democratic redistribution of policy-making capability while serving their political masters.

For critical theory to have widespread and intended practical effect in resisting patterns of governance that frustrate democratic access, it must consciously shape the practitioner's daily work. Agger (1992) argues for a "lifeworld-grounded critical theory" that "attempts to identify resistances and transformations already taking place in the quotidian worlds in which all of us live" (p. 219). The practitioner who chooses to adopt such a view of critical theory as a guide to action serves as an "interpreter" of professional knowledge for citizens and governing bodies (Box, 1992), and as a "communitarian facilitator," shifting "attention from the 'distal' environment of the clientele to the 'proximate' environment of the face-to-face work group" (Catron & Hammond, 1992, p. 246).

This "interpreter/facilitator" role of the public professional within critical theory uses powerful, yet indirect, techniques. It contains, simultaneously, an element of the professional expertise espoused by the reform movement of the early twentieth century and an activist concern for equalizing democratic access to the power of governance. This role does not require a general readjustment of relationships between professionals and governmental institutions, nor does it place demands for change on the American social system in advance of doing its work. Instead, it promotes rational-democratic decision making wherever a public professional is ready to assume the associated challenges and risks.

It may seem like a hopeless project to bring control of complex modern social systems, with their experts and purposive-rational structures, within reach of those who are governed. In contemporary social systems, "democracy is like nearly everything else we do; it is a form of collaboration of ignorant people and experts" (Schattschneider, 1960, p. 134). However, as public professionals may paradoxically gain effectiveness by giving away authority, they may also be returning, paradoxically, to an earlier vision of the American public in affirming the value of enlightenment and emancipation. As Thomas Jefferson said, "wherever the people are well informed they can be trusted with their own government," and, "if we think them [that is, the people] not enlightened enough to exercise their control with a wholesome discretion, the remedy is not to take it from them, but to inform their discretion by education" (Matthews, 1984, p. 88).

— 5 —

Pragmatic Discourse and Administrative Legitimacy

Legitimacy, the place of public administration in governance, always has been a concern in American society. Responses to this concern have included efforts to control bureaucracy by defining what it should do, to free it from control by elevating its status in relation to other branches of government, and to confine it to microlevel, market-like management techniques. The discourse theory of O.C. McSwite, based on pragmatism, suggests that governmental legitimacy in America may be revived by shifting from an emphasis on the public administrator's role in directing agencies to thinking about how administrators may assist in creating community through collaboration with citizens. This chapter offers a critique and extension of McSwite's work based in part on critical theory, arguing that to recover administrative legitimacy through collaborative discourse it may be necessary to recognize and respond to the nature of the liberal-capitalist political environment.

Public administration plays a significant role in governance, not only on the implementation side of the continuum of public action but on the decision-making side as well. Although this has been recognized for some

From *American Review of Public Administration*, vol. 32, no. 1 (March 2002): 20–39. Copyright © 2002 Sage Publications, Inc. Reprinted with permission.

time (Waldo, 1980), it always has been in question in American society, in which people are wary of control by government in general and by powerful officials and unelected administrators in particular. One way this attitude is reflected in the literature of public administration is a concern with the "legitimacy" of career, unelected administrators in a democratic society.

There have been several responses to this concern. One is to control bureaucracy by setting boundaries around what public administrators should do (Finer, 1941; Gruber, 1987; Lowi, 1993; Stewart, 1992) or confining public administration to a traditional, constitutional framework (Lynn, 2001; Rohr, 1978). Another is to elevate administration from its position as tool of elected legislators to the status of equal institutional partner (Spicer & Terry, 1993; Wamsley et al., 1987). A third response is to reassert the separation of politics and administration through the application of economic models (Moe, 1984) focusing on the microlevel perspective of public bureaucracy and management as a starting point, giving relatively little attention to the larger, macrolevel position of public administration in a democratic polity (Kirlin, 1996).

These responses to the concern with legitimacy have the matter of control at their core, either public desire to assert greater control over bureaucracy or administrative desire to break free from control. The third response, the application of economic models in the public sphere, is an understandable movement toward instrumental technique and away from the discussion of substantive issues. It is understandable because this is a time of political pressure to give the appearance of efficiency (Miller & Nunemaker, 1999), offering instant gratification to a public with a short attention span and a skeptical view of government (Fox & Miller, 1995; King & Stivers, 1998). Nevertheless, it can be as important to consider "social and value conflicts in the larger society" (Ventriss, 2000, p. 502) as it is to focus on "economic and methodistic approaches" (p. 515).

Against the backdrop of this emphasis on control of bureaucracy, an alternative or supplemental notion is offered of administrative legitimacy. It does not require abandoning the concept of control, which in some form will likely always be with us. This alternative view is that administrative legitimacy is the product of understandings created by participants in public discourse. It is pragmatic in looking toward the future and depending on social interaction to create nonfoundational "edifying first-order narratives" (Rorty, 1991, p. 212) as working hypotheses. It also has a critical edge because public administrators, in facilitating discourse and sharing knowledge of alternative practices, may give citizens opportunities to take public will formation in new and different directions that challenge the status quo.

"Discourse theory" (Farmer, 1995; Fox & Miller, 1995; McSwite, 1997) is emerging in public administration as a way to recapture a sense of public administration outside the narrow confines of management technique and efficiency. It seeks to free citizens and administrators from reified, theoretical preconceptions and institutional constraints, allowing them to re-create themselves and their institutional arrangements in current discourse settings. This idea is not new, but the focus on discourse and the application of theoretical constructs from pragmatism, postmodernism, and critical theory present new ways to think about an old problem.

The alternative notion of legitimacy discussed here shifts attention away from legitimacy in the context of control of bureaucracy, moving it toward conceiving of administrative legitimacy in the context of discourse with citizens and the potential to release new understandings of social conditions and possibilities for collective action. The following narrative reviews some of the discourse theory being discussed in public administration, then focuses on the work of O.C. McSwite, which is based on pragmatism. A possible extension of McSwite's work is offered, drawing in part on a critical analysis of what citizens know and what information administrators can provide. The article concludes by arguing that in certain discourse settings, the legitimate purpose of administration is discovered not by predetermined roles but through collaborative action.

Discourse theory in public administration is the work of several authors, so generalization requires care. The work of Cynthia McSwain and Orion White (individually and writing as O.C. McSwite) and of Charles Fox and Hugh Miller focuses on the discourse process, and David John Farmer has worked from multiple theoretical perspectives to offer a broad view of interrelationships in governance systems. Discourse may include a variety of settings for collaboration among citizens, administrators, and elected representatives. It may involve communication between individuals or in small or large groups, it may occur over significant periods of time, and it may include combinations of media such as meetings and electronic communication.

Although authors differ even in areas of commonality, themes among discourse theorists include antifoundational resistance to metanarratives (disbelief in the primacy and objectivity of any single theory or description of phenomena), a constructivist view of knowledge (reality as the product of human thought rather than given by the external world), and the search for free and uncoerced communication in open discourse settings. In these settings, people are able to discuss what to do next, relatively unfettered by the values and predictability that institutional or functional theory would impose. According to McSwite (2000, p. 55), people create themselves in the interactive process of working together on problems, whereas for functionalists (and classical liberals in political theory), individuals come to the discourse process as predetermined packages of interests or as, to exaggerate the point, "robots operated by values."

Beyond these nonrationalist (not irrationalist), postmodern thoughts, there is divergence in discourse theorists' conceptualizations of the nature of the problems that lead to prescriptions for discourse and in the substance of those prescriptions. Fox and Miller (1995) framed the current social situation in terms of a postmodern "thinning" of reality in which terms and images are increasingly separated from "authentic" discourse, and a genuine sense of community can only be found in small, localized enclaves. This makes "democratic will formation and policy discourse increasingly problematic" (p. 7). Fox and Miller were concerned that the *"representative democratic accountability feedback loop* model of democracy" (p. 4), in which aggregated citizen preferences are pooled to elect representatives who appoint administrators to carry out their policies, is an inadequate and undemocratic way to govern. Evidence of this includes, among other things, the manipulation of public opinion, the feeding frenzy of Washington lobbyists, and the control of local governance by economic interests (pp. 16–17).

Fox and Miller (1995) argued that not everyone will participate in discourse on every issue. To expect that they could, or would wish to, was to Fox and Miller an unreasonable communitarian premise, colorfully described as a way to "bypass the masters of ill-begotten political superordination and make common cause with the citizens themselves" (p. 33). Fox and Miller recognized that "the powerful can ensure that certain classes of people are excluded from the debate" (p. 10), so the opposite of everyone participating, decision making by a select few, is not acceptable on democratic grounds. Thus, we find ourselves in a situation in which some people participate, and it is a matter of creating for them something like Jürgen Habermas's "ideal speech" situation. Drawing from the work of Hannah Arendt, Fox and Miller characterized public discourse as "agonistic," meaning that discussion will be argumentative as people "try to resolve what to do next" (p. 11). To provide "discipline" for the discourse process, Fox and Miller suggested the use of four "warrants" for entry into a discourse setting: sincerity, situation-regarding intentionality, willing attention, and substantive contribution. Public administrators play a proactive role (as per

Harmon, 1981) in creating possibilities for discourse, but this is not easy, because "life is more complicated for the public administrator who peeks out from the protective umbrella of neutral competence where technical criteria guided action" (Fox & Miller, 1995, p. 157).

Farmer's (2000b) work covers much ground at a level of analysis broader than the discourse setting. In writing of discourses that leave out "important elements of what it is to be human" (p. 81), Farmer noted that "the discourse that constitutes the economic or capitalist machine, designed to optimize profits, is an example" (p. 82). On the smaller scale of public administration, Farmer's concept of "antiadministration" shares much with other discourse theorists and offers a wide-ranging assessment of public administration and postmodernism. To the extent that antiadministration were to be implemented, the political-governmental system would be more fluid, tentative, and open to a diversity of views. Administrators would prefer building citizens' sense of community to creating ever larger rational-instrumental bureaucracies. Farmer's (1995, p. 244) "postmodern administrator is likely to be one who is skilled in practicing and developing the implications of antiadministration," including "an openness to the 'other,'" which involves antiauthoritarian administration, a service attitude, open decision making, avoiding imposing bureaucratic attitudes and practices on communities, and "micropolitics in the form of local community action" (p. 245).

Also, antiadministration involves resisting established authority: Citizens or administrators might engage in acts of "refusal" against "the administered life" (Farmer, 2000a). The language of refusal comes from critical theorist Herbert Marcuse (1964, pp. 63–64, 254–257). This is the side of Marcuse that "champions individual rebellion" (Kellner, 1984, p. 373), as compared to large-scale social action, though both include forms of emancipation. Parenthetically, compare Farmer's concern about the administered society to Tocqueville's thoughts about the administered democracy, containing people:

> alike and equal, constantly circling around in pursuit of the petty and banal pleasures with which they glut their souls. . . . Over this kind of men stands an immense, protective power which is alone responsible for securing their enjoy-ment and watching over their fate. That power is absolute, thoughtful of detail, orderly, provident, and gentle.
>
> Thus it daily makes the exercise of free choice less useful and rarer, restricts the activity of free will within a narrower compass, and little by little robs each citizen of the proper use of his own faculties. (Tocqueville, 1969, p. 692)

To McSwite (1997, pp. 43–52), the legitimacy of control consists of the idea that governance means a process by which legislators and administrators create and carry out "policies"; that is to say, fixed, systematic, standardized, programmatic prescriptions that treat everyone alike. These policies and programs are steered by the legislator or administrator operating as a "guiding consciousness," seeking realistic and efficient outcomes. To keep such a system running, citizens must be content to turn over the process to elected leaders and their hired professionals, "leaving our participation in governance ultimately to the crude devices of elections and interest groups" (p. 51). This is the "man-of-reason" phenomenon, in which certain people assert control to maximize rational, cost-efficient results, employees are to be held accountable, and policy outcomes are reasoned and consistent.

In McSwite's (1997) narrative, this situation is a product of the misfounding of the field of public administration. Centralized, interest-based government built on instrumental reason ("federalist" government) has been the winner in a competition with the opposing tradition of dialogue, localism, and cooperative relationship in community ("antifederalist" government). Such a misfounding requires some degree of intentionality and willingness to use power to exclude subjectivity and relationship from public governance. To McSwite (1998a), the situation is worsening as people respond to the seeming failure of "citizen participation" to address the problems in the social system by adopting measures of "technological control" (p. 273). McSwite was concerned that what "economic rationalism" as practiced by classical liberals "is going to give us is a world that brings us all under the domination of the efficiency principle, as measured by the attainment of the lowest price for everything" (p. 277).

McSwite's (1997) discourse prescription consists of a "process theory" termed *collaborative pragmatism,* drawn from the spirit of "cooperative community, benevolence, and social coherence" (p. 16). It draws inspiration from the work of pragmatist Mary Parker Follett ([1918] 1998), such as her book *The New State: Group Organization the Solution of Popular Government,* in which she advocated "group process" as an alternative to individualism, parties and interests, and representative, ballot-box democracy. With Michael Harmon's (1981) "action theory," McSwite's discourse process emphasizes the face-to-face encounter and the search for agreement on what to do next rather than acting out preconceived roles. Collaborative pragmatism means that people join together to seek agreement on action, unconstrained by history, values, and reified, institutional structures. Instead of behaving as individualized packets of predetermined interests, consistent with the standard liberal model of citizenship and human nature, people find themselves transformed by the interactive discourse setting, the encounter with the "other." This process of citizens finding meaning in joint action is contrasted with the dominant theme of capitalist democracy as an efficient way to exploit the ecosystem to produce "the greatest degree of gratification at the lowest price" (McSwite, 1997, p. 274). McSwite (1998a, p. 277) hoped that collaborative pragmatism would help solve "the pressing problem of social diversity and ethnic (in the broadest sense of the term) conflict."

The Limits of Theory

New work by authors joining the discussion of discourse includes that of Arthur Sementelli and Richard Hezog (2000) on discourse theory and budgeting; Frank Scott (2000) on rational instrumentalism versus nonrational human relationships in discourse theory; Patricia Patterson (2000) on whether the warrants of discourse exclude silenced voices; and Cheryl Simrell King (2000) on rational versus nonrational approaches, including storytelling and narrative. Also, other public administration writers have used discourse-related themes in addressing questions of citizen involvement in governance. These include Camilla Stivers (1994, 2000a, 2000b), King and Stivers (1998), Lisa Zanetti (1997), and Richard Box (1995, 1998).

One should be careful, however, about one's normative and epistemological premises in joining the stream of developing thought in discourse. McSwite (1998b) contrasted their version of discourse theory with the "new normativists," including authors such as Philip Selznick, Benjamin Barber, Michael Sandel, and Anthony Giddens. McSwite agreed with these writers that values are subjective and cannot be precisely defined, but did not agree that "ambiguities that arise around them can be worked out within the safe context of the authoritative (legitimate) leadership and processes that institutions afford" (p. 379). To McSwite, the purpose of discourse theory is to introduce into the public discussion ideas from outside current understandings of institutional structures and practices rather than to accept them as normative grounding.

The question of epistemology is as sensitive as that of normative orientation. Kenneth Hansen (1998) suggested that Fox and Miller's (1995) warrants for discourse are subject to the "eye of the beholder" problem; that is, they are a matter of subjective interpretation and so do not help identify when discourse settings are working properly. To correct this problem, Hansen suggested instead three "empirical referents of discourse":

inclusion (coalition building, the acceptance of outsiders, and community outreach activities), self-regulation (empowerment by election of leaders; the negotiation of operating norms, rules, and procedures; and techniques such as roundtables instead of podiums or the availability of toll-free numbers or e-mail addresses that encourage multidirectional instead of monological communication), and policy outputs (the development of organizations to take action, adequate funding, completed strategic plans, and evidence of implementation).

Published with Hansen's (1998) article were responses by Miller (1998) and White (1998). White was concerned that Hansen's empiricism leads back to failed attempts of the past to get citizens to participate in governance without changing the system itself, so that true discourse, as a transformative process, never takes place. Discourse is "synergistic and evocative" (White, 1998, p. 473), and "when discourse takes off and gains the life of its own that it must have if it is to work, it cannot be comprehended in objective or any other conscious terms" (p. 475). Interestingly, White viewed Fox and Miller's (1995) warrants as barely avoiding sliding down the slippery slope of traditional empiricism that claimed Hansen.

Miller (1998) critiqued Hansen's (1998) choices of empirical referents, noting that the election of leaders could as easily degrade substantive discussion of issues as it could produce greater democracy and, contra Hansen's claim that valid discourse must produce policy outcomes, "sometimes, preventing action would be the better indication that democracy had taken place" (Miller, 1998, p. 463). But, Miller's primary point of disagreement was that Hansen had set up supposedly objective criteria of measurement for situations that might successfully be described as they happen but cannot be predicted and controlled if they are to succeed. Miller took care to note he was not arguing against research that would document the characteristics of discourse processes, but that by attempting to predetermine what discourse should be about, Hansen fell into the trap of thinking that truth can be "achieved at an ivory-tower distance from the participants." Miller would have felt better about Hansen's effort if it had been constructed so that "the results of his research were turned back over to the community as a substantive contribution to the discourse" (p. 464).

These responses to an attempt to draw discourse into the mainstream of traditional public administration empiricism help in understanding the assumptions underlying discourse theory as introduced by the authors discussed here. Their discourse process is not predetermined and constrained by rules and outcome expectations. It is not something to be "gotten through" to be able to get on with implementing a program that was going to happen anyway, nor is it a way, via strategic planning, to discover a single path for action. From the point of view of those of us sympathetic to the discourse perspective, these are good things to learn. However, they are also cautionary lessons because the sphere of acceptable conceptualization in discourse theory seems to have limits.

The Usefulness of Pragmatism

Much attention has been given in the literature to Fox and Miller's (1995) use of Habermasian warrants for discourse. The intent here is to more fully explore the work of McSwite, in part because it is based on pragmatism, which is important to knowledge and action in the United States, and in part because it presents an especially strong argument against objectivity, certainty, and traditional perspectives on public policy formulation and implementation. One needs to examine whether it is possible to preserve pragmatism's focus on the future (rather than ideas and structures from the past) while acknowledging certain social conditions and the desire one might feel to change them.

This is a friendly probing of McSwite's discourse theory. I am sympathetic to White's (1998, p. 471) comment that introduction of discourse theory into public administration is "immensely auspicious, perhaps its salvation from the threat of being completely overtaken by a market-based rational-choice brand of thought." The discussion in this section compares McSwite's analysis of the challenge we face and the history that brought us here, with their prescription for change: collaborative pragmatism. The argument is that the prescription may not be sufficient to meet the challenge and that an extension of the collaborative pragmatism model could help remedy the problem.

McSwite has portrayed contemporary public governance set in a technological, market-driven environment resulting from the victory of forces of wealth, power, and centralization. The discourse process of collaborative pragmatism seems to float free in its own time and space, largely untouched by the grubbiness of self-interest, control by elites for their own benefit, and the impact on consciousness of a liberal-capitalist society that rewards people for accepting the consumerist economic machine as the highest good.

McSwite (2000, pp. 47–48) contrasted their utopian view of attaining completely transparent communication with the view of Camilla Stivers, who, according to McSwite, is interested in finding ways to accommodate discourse to existing patterns of power so that administrators and citizens can form better relationships. Many people would find themselves with McSwite in hoping for "ideal" communication. They also might think that action toward that ideal requires attention to the daily reality of people's lives and what is needed to give them an opportunity to engage in authentic discourse. To adapt the metaphor Miller (1998) used in his reply to Hansen (1998), for the tail of discourse to wag the dog of public governance, it may need to acknowledge the gritty nature of the dog's environment.

Collaborative pragmatism is based on philosophical pragmatism, which has been criticized for being passive and instrumental in relation to surrounding social phenomena. Pragmatists make no secret of the "instrumental" nature of their philosophy, which, according to William James (1907, pp. 54–55), involves "the attitude of looking away from first things, principles, 'categories,' supposed necessities; and of looking towards last things, fruits, consequences, facts." In this search for the consequences of theories and actions, James asked a question and made an assertion: "In what respects would the world be different if this alternative or that were true? If I can find nothing that would become different, then the alternative has no sense" (p. 48). In this way, pragmatism is the reverse of rationalism, assuming no position in advance of investigation and serving a purely instrumental role. As James put it, pragmatism "does not stand for any special results. It is a method only" (p. 51). James quoted the Italian philosopher Papini in noting that pragmatism "lies in the midst of our theories, like a corridor in a hotel. Innumerable chambers open out of it" (p. 54). To James, then, pragmatism appeared not as a solution to problems, but as "a program for more work, and more particularly as an indication of the ways in which existing realities may be *changed. Theories thus become instruments, not answers to enigmas, in which we can rest.* We don't lie back upon them, we move forward, and, on occasion, make nature over again by their aid" (p. 53).

Lewis Mumford (1950a; 1950b) characterized the instrumental nature of pragmatist John Dewey's philosophy as a weakness, acquiescence to the status quo, a triumph of technique joined with lack of vision. To Mumford, pragmatism was born of the American experience in throwing off the faded rationalism of the past and creating a new society through science and experimentation. Mumford saw this as good as far as it goes, but there is always the question of what values are being served and how pragmatists choose the values they advocate.

The instrumental nature of pragmatism has not kept pragmatists from arguing for views of society that imply the need for change. C. Wright Mills believed that Dewey ignored differences between people and held a naive view of democracy belied by the actualities of social conflict and power relationships (Campbell, 1995, pp. 225–265). Dewey thought that social problems could be addressed by getting people together in "cooperative inquiry" to discover what should be done. To Mills, "a more accurate analysis of our circumstances realizes that one person's or group's good is often another's evil" (Campbell, 1995, p. 243), so that "a more realistic analysis would be to see social action as struggle" (p. 241). Nevertheless, according to Campbell, Dewey did not ignore social conditions and believed that "people have been systematically miseducated and propagandized, alienated in their working lives and exploited in their economic relations" (p. 227).

Contemporary pragmatist Richard Rorty (1999) has addressed the question of whether the pragmatic approach to knowledge is useful in solving social problems by suggesting a separation between philosophy and social action. Rorty defended liberal society as the best way to allow people freedom to invent themselves as they choose, but he also wrote of the struggle between rich and poor and of the "global overclass which makes all the major economic decisions" (p. 233). Rorty identified the "central political questions" as follows: "How can the working class in a democratic society use the power of the ballot to prevent the capitalists from immiserating the proletariat, while still encouraging business enterprise? How can the state be a countervailing power, one which will prevent all the wealth winding up in the hands of an economic oligarchy, without creating bureaucratic stagnation?" (pp. 232–233).

Discussion of the instrumental limitations of pragmatism appears in recent work in public administration. Lisa Zanetti and Adrian Carr (2000) noted that critical theorists have found pragmatism to be limited by its failure to understand the effects of its sociohistorical context and the language it uses, language that "itself is a vehicle of and for ideology." Thus, a sort of "social amnesia" takes hold, in which "we are left with a received view of social realities rather than what might he an alternative vision" (p. 444). This parallels Herbert Marcuse's (1964, p. 174) notion of "purged language," that is language that has been "purged not only of its 'unorthodox' vocabulary, but also of the means of expressing any other contents than those furnished to the individuals by their society." Zanetti and Carr (2000, p. 448) believed that philosophy "has a responsibility—an obligation, even—to get its hands dirty in the real world of politics and power." Thus, "it is precisely for this reason that we argue many contemporary pragmatists ultimately fall short" (p. 448).

Discourse theorists sometimes seem to hedge issues of power in society, institutions, and discourse settings. This may be because power is equated with reified institutional formations, conflicting with the idea of discourse existing in an open field of possibilities uncontrolled by the past. As McSwite (1998b, pp. 379–380) put it, "discourse is premised on the idea that the status quo may indeed be the best or all that we have; however, that was then, this is now." This makes sense as an ideal, but citizens and public-service practitioners often encounter discourse settings that involve ideologies, agendas, and on occasion ignorance or upsetting behavior. It can be a challenge to find ways to work with the baggage people bring to a discourse setting, accepting it but enabling participants to form new understandings on the basis of moving beyond where they were when they entered the process.

One might wonder whether the idea of discourse could become so rarefied and divorced from the lifeworld that it can no longer be used to think in a practical way about daily work in discourse settings. Miller (1998) noted that Hansen (1998) erred by moving deductively to supposedly objective measures, skipping over the subjective, inductive human content that constitutes discourse. White (1998, p. 472) described the problem as believing "that differences in perception can be resolved definitively by the device of objective indicators grounded in compelling evidence." Hansen (1998, p. 451) wrote that discourse can be "objectively observed," but from a postpositivist perspective, an awareness of the untenability of that position has been around for some time (Lincoln & Guba, 1985). Observers may try to be unobtrusive and report faithfully what they think has been seen and heard, but they bring with them a full complement of human subjectivity.

To those who have spent time in public discourse settings, it is clear enough that one must be cautious about generalizing. From one discourse setting to the next, the mixture of external influences and the personalities and emotional and intellectual characteristics of participants produces seemingly infinite combinations of action and result. Each discourse setting involves unique people and phenomena, and surrounding institutions and practices can be changed as new understandings emerge during discourse.

On the other hand, experience in these settings reveals patterns that can be communicated to others as scholarly writing or as information useful for practitioners. At any point in time, people can identify common features of collaborative work, using them to guide their own research and practice. Discourse is not so mysterious that it is beyond human ability to create partial, tentative, dynamic descriptions to aid in understanding. People come to a discourse setting with some awareness of the social context, with intellectual precommitments, and with "aspects of the human condition that come before language—things such as feelings, emotions, the unconscious, unthinking habituation, background, socialization, historical experience, patterns, and practices that have become second nature" (Miller, 1998, p. 465).

At some point, agreement on what to do, however tentative, may emerge from a discourse setting, causing certain actions to be taken by public employees. Calling an agreed-on course of action a policy or program may make it seem final or coercive because it takes on a perceived identity outside the process in which it was created, becoming a fixed mandate beyond further discussion. For two reasons, it might be useful to use alternative language or rehabilitate the language we have. One reason is to share an understanding of what occurs when citizens reach agreement on what they want done. The other is to reorient the meaning of the words used to describe discourse outcomes so it is clear that they are malleable, dynamic constructions, experiments in public governance.

Collaboration and Critical Thought

With the above exploration of potential limitations of the theoretical basis of McSwite's discourse setting, it will be useful to think further about the place of discourse in allowing people to recognize and achieve a desirable future. Collaborative pragmatism, if fully realized, might appear much like communitarian prescriptions. As noted earlier, it is akin to the approach of Mary Parker Follett ([1918] 1998) in the early twentieth century. It is also similar to the "dialogical communitarianism" of Elizabeth Frazer and Nicola Lacey (1993), which steers an interpretivist midcourse between liberal individualism and the potential oppressiveness of group conformity in communitarianism. Like some other feminist authors (Elshtain, 1981; Fraser, 1989), Frazer and Lacey worried that predefining certain issues as inappropriate for public discussion preserves inequities built into the status quo.

McSwite (1998a) wrote that liberals fear discourse processes because they may degenerate into conflict and threaten individual rights. In commenting on McSwite's work, liberal Kenneth Ruscio (1998) imagined citizens, in public discourse, questioning existing legal-institutional arrangements and discussing issues that liberals would prefer to keep private. He feared that this could result in "forsaking of reason and the enactment of public discourse without boundaries, based more on therapeutic self-realization than careful deliberation about the public (as opposed to the personal) good" (p. 271). Consistent with their premise that reason is used by those who wish to limit public discourse to control others, McSwite (1998a, p. 278) responded that "if we have relationship, we do not need reason." Mary Parker Follett ([1918] 1998, p. 189) captured this view of the public-private question more than eight decades ago: "We are now beginning to recognize more and more clearly that the work we do, the conditions of that work, the houses in which we live, the water we drink, the food we eat, the opportunities for bringing up our children, that in fact the whole area of our daily life should constitute politics. There is no line where the life of the home ends and the life of the city begins."

McSwite retains optimism about the possibilities for collaborative action, hoping that it may help with questions of diversity and ethnic conflict. In part, McSwite does so by assuming that the current technicist period may end, allowing the traditional, "antifederalist," collaborative-republican model of society to reassert itself against the federalist-liberal view of citizens as independent bearers of rights. However, this optimistic assumption may be on shaky ground. The constitutional debate involved a range of issues, but Gordon Wood (1969, pp. 484–485) wrote that it "can best be understood as a social one. . . . The quarrel was fundamentally one between aristocracy and democracy." Wood portrayed the conflict of Federalists and Anti-Federalists as between an elite advocating centralization in favor of order and property and the mass of citizens defending a heterogeneous, populist localism and the right to develop free from control by their social "betters."

Both Federalists and Anti-Federalists spoke and wrote of republican civic virtue. Richard Sinopoli (1992) argued that they considered it a secondary value within the context of liberal concern with securing individual rights from violation by others and by the government. According to Sinopoli, the Anti-Federalists, in defending ideas such as "the powers of local government and the enhancement of democratic participation through such policies as rotation in office, recall, and short terms of office—were liberals when it came to defining first principles" (p. 7). These things were intended "first and foremost to check the power lust and acquisitive desires of rulers. . . . The essential purpose of government for most Anti-Federalists, as much as for Publius, was the preservation of rights conceived as natural rights" (p. 7). Antifederalist, localist thinking remains vital and important in America, but Saul Cornell (1999, p. 306) wrote that it is "capable of producing both libertarianism and consensual communitarianism." Thus, it can be used to support liberal individualism as well as cooperative democracy. Overall, it appears that antifederalism contains elements of republican virtue, but republicanism may not be a long-suppressed central societal principle waiting to be reborn when the time is right.

McSwite (1997) noted that democratic impulses cropped up at various times following the Federalist "victory," including during the Progressive era. Early in the twentieth century, Mary Parker Follett was part of the movement to foster democratic decision making by creating community centers, places where citizens could meet to develop ideas and initiate reform (Mattson, 1998, pp. 87–104). Follett did not want merely to encourage citizens to participate by expressing opinions on public affairs. Instead, through organizing at the neighborhood level and problem solving with others, people would come to believe it "is not that I serve my neighborhood, my city, my nation, but that by this service I become my neighborhood, my city, my nation" (Follett, [1918] 1998, p. 242).

Follett's vision of progressive improvement through cooperative citizen action was not sustainable. By the 1920s, community centers had become recreation-oriented places controlled by professional social workers (Mattson, 1998, pp. 120–125). Instead of face-to-face cooperative dialogue with neighbors, "few citizens seemed concerned about a public or common good; rather, they seemed (during that so-called Jazz Age of the 1920s) obsessed with satisfying their private needs through the market of consumer goods and a culture of consumption" (p. 126). Walter Lippmann (1922) argued that the public had become a passive mass to be manipulated by elites. A parallel can be found today in the perceived decline of civic culture (Putnam, 2000) and fragmentation of society into an individualism of self-centered "lifestyle politics" (Bennett, 1998).

Judging from this limited examination of history and social collaboration, it seems that people have not always been ready for long-term commitment to building a self-governing society. As one examines perspectives of society and the desire for collaborative social action, over time one finds continuity in the problem of creating cooperative democracy in a liberal-capitalist setting. In the early twentieth century, John Dewey's critics believed that whatever his personal democratic values, his idea of cooperative inquiry was insufficient given the conditions in society. McSwite's collaborative pragmatism might be in the same situation, but it could be argued that this does not matter because the point is to get beyond man-of-reason legitimacy of control and allow people to do as they wish with governance of their collective community. This argument assumes several things that may be problematic, including that people know that there is a problem that needs to be solved, that they know how to bring interested people together, that they have access to the information required for informed discussion of the questions before them, and that their process will not be interrupted by the actions of elites who feel their interests to be threatened. These are strong assumptions. Critical theorists would suggest that people often are not fully aware of the problems they face and the action options open to them, that they may be denied access to the information needed to develop a clear understanding of their situation, and that they could be ignored or in some way suppressed if their actions threaten economic or political interests (Box, 1995, 1998; Logan & Molotch, 1987).

One can identify a continuum of perceived need for collective action. At one end, perceived need for change is not an issue, either because things seem fine as they are or because there is no hope for a vision of change to succeed. At the other end, it is believed to be time for people to oppose the status quo and work toward a utopian vision. At the not-an-issue end of the continuum may be found satisfaction with the liberal-capitalist order, which provides an "accommodation" between property rights and personal rights (Bowles & Gintis, 1986), allowing people to shape their lives with a minimum of interference from others. Also at this end is a skeptical postmodernism, perceiving fragmentation, chaos, ambiguity, and resignation so deep that "in this period no social or political project is worthy of commitment" (Rosenau, 1992, p. 15).

At the time-for-action end of the continuum is found the critical theory project of enlightening people so that they may discover the true nature of their condition, becoming "emancipated" and capable of shaping their lives free from illusions of well-being created by contemporary society (Geuss, 1981). Communitarianism (Sandel, 1996) holds an intermediate position on this continuum, as does Rorty's (1999) pragmatism, offering melioration of some of the grosser abuses of the liberal-capitalist order, and McSwite's collaborative pragmatism, which offers hope of transcending it. Also in this intermediate area is a critical theory ready to engage in daily politics but mindful of the limitations imposed on universalist emancipatory visions by a political arena that "is increasingly dominated by the rituals of pseudodemocracy" (Agger, 1992, p. 305). This position retains hope for the future despite the failure of broad social change in the face of the dominance of the capitalist order, resorting instead to isolated acts of resistance such as Marcuse's (1964) idea of refusing to participate in aspects of the dominant society.

For discourse theory to facilitate citizen efforts toward self-governance, it may be necessary to acknowledge that social problems are intertwined with economic and political conditions and people's beliefs and also that collective action may be resisted by those who benefit from the status quo.

This need not mean assuming (as with the "strong" version of critical theory) that there is a "real" world of freedom and democracy underlying the shadow appearances of the daily lifeworld, nor should it mean fantasizing about (in the manner of classical liberalism) a one-time, permanent settlement in the interrelationship of citizens, government, and powerful groups in the form of constitutions, laws, institutions, polices, or ideas about what is public and what is private. The acknowledgment of extant conditions in the social environment should be able to coexist with discourse theory's antifoundational openness and orientation toward the future.

Conclusion: Administrative Legitimacy

Given the potential uses of power in discourse settings and the technicist orientation of public administration accompanying what McSwite calls its "misfounding," reconceptualizing legitimacy as the product of collaborative discussion instead of control is not easy. Discourse theory informed by awareness of the societal barriers to open discussion helps in this reconceptualization. If legitimacy is primarily a matter of debate over the role of bureaucracy, public administrators who facilitate citizen awareness of existing practices and potential alternatives need protection from the charge of acting outside their prescribed sphere of discretion. They may accidentally stir the hornet's nest of classical liberal worry about unruly citizens and direct democracy, traceable in the United States back to the colonial and founding eras (Wood, 1969). In so doing, they may find themselves accused of endangering the stability of hallowed, reified public institutions and being in league with academicians who "in promoting community and civic empowerment, barely acknowledge the constitutional role of legislatures, courts, and executive departments" (Lynn, 2001, pp. 154–155).

The literature of discourse and citizenship offers several models of administrative action consistent with viewing legitimacy as the understanding that arises in a discourse process between citizens and practitioners about administrative action. Such understandings often are contested rather than consensual and are contingent on the needs of a particular time and set of issues rather than fixed and long lasting. Fox and Miller's administrator is proactive in seeking democratic will formation, Farmer's "antiadministration" administrator minimizes bureaucratic control and opens governance to the community, McSwite's administrator avoids acting as a "man of reason," and Stivers's administrator is a responsive listener. Adding critical theory to the discourse process, Zanetti (1997) drew inspiration for her model of administrative action in part from Antonio Gramsci and Brazilian critical theorist Paulo Freire. Her administrators act in a critical, emancipatory mode, teaching citizens how to articulate concerns and implement change. There are similarities in this model to Box's (1998) "helper" administrator, who gives away knowledge and control to help citizens self-govern. Both models are built on a critical analysis of power and knowledge, assuming that in a liberal-capitalist society, to fully self-govern, citizens must be given information that has been kept from them, and they must be provided a discourse setting that allows them to use this knowledge. Zanetti's model is more forthright in pressing an emancipatory administrative intent that shapes the character of the discourse process.

None of these models of action is easy or risk-free, nor are they appropriate for all public-service practitioners in all situations. However, for some, there are opportunities to move away from standard models of legitimacy to become part of a joint process, with citizens, of constructing a different future. Examples could include a staff member tasked with organizing neighborhood residents to identify problems and solutions, the administrator of a community-oriented policing project, a land-use planner who serves as a staff member for citizen problem-solving sessions, and an administrator who finds the right time to suggest that a governing body open the governance process by forming new citizen committees or boards.

Choices made by administrators about information, mode of presentation, and process may constrain collaborative citizen action instead of facilitating it. Farmer (1995, p. 245), quoting Michel Foucault, cautioned that it is wise to be aware of "the fascism in us all." Citizens may not always be able on their own to initiate and sustain collaborative discourse. As Lippmann wrote in 1922, citizens cannot be expected to be "omnicompetent" in obtaining sufficient knowledge to participate meaningfully in a public dialogue. This leaves the field open for experts, politicians, and publicists to guide public opinion with simplification and slogan, creating a "pseudoenvironment" in which leaders are free to go their chosen direction. When a public administrator steps into the space between citizens who need knowledge and the opportunity to use it and a political setting that resists change, a healthy response might include reflective self-questioning, because, as John Dewey (1927, pp. 205–206) put it, "Rule by an economic class may be disguised from the masses; rule by experts could not be covered up. It could be made to work only if the intellectuals became the willing tools of big economic interests. Otherwise they would have to ally themselves with the masses, and that implies, once more, a share in government by the latter."

For the public administrator, the power, institutions, and other features that inhabit discourse settings are not only pesky reifications. In the administrator's office are laws, regulations, policies, budgets, personnel rules and labor agreements, and paper and electronic files dealing with official business and so forth. These things may be regarded as hard demarcations of a role or alternatively as a cross-sectional glimpse at an unfolding process reflecting the attitudes, opinions, and preferences of citizens, the administrator's bureaucratic and elected superiors, interest groups, and the media. Theories of contingency and social construction are not new in political thought. Thomas Jefferson believed, as part of "radical democracy," that all laws and constitutions should be terminated every nineteen years (the length of a generation) so that people could re-create their society (Matthews, 1984, pp. 22, 126). This sense of limitless change is echoed in Chantal Mouffe's (1996, p. 11) comment that "in Derrida's words, democracy will always be 'to come,' traversed by undecidability and for ever keeping open its element of promise."

Much of the discussion of legitimacy in American public administration has revolved around the Constitution and the relationship of executive branch agencies to Congress, the courts, and organized interests. However, of the more than 87,000 units of government in the United States, this Constitution-based dialogue has immediate relevance to only 1 (the nation), less direct relevance to 50 others (the states), and indirect relevance to all the rest. Most public employees, elected officials, and citizens encounter discourse settings not in an environment constrained by lofty concern with constitutional intent, but instead by concern with local history, personalities, economics, and politics. To the extent that national-level structural or legal issues impinge at this level, they do so more as external factors than as fundamental principles of legitimacy (for instance, case law related to police procedures, Forest Service policy on working with state and local fire control agencies, restrictions on the use of grant monies, and so on). For most people, the factors that affect discourse settings are more immediate and close at hand. This does not mean that barriers to effective discourse are insignificant, only that they are sometimes closer to human scale and more accessible to change than is commonly thought.

It is important to distinguish between two ways of thinking about society, institutions, and other elements of a discourse context. One is to imagine them as fixed and authoritative, a stable and restrictive foundation for human action. The other is to think of them as malleable, useful or harmful, simple or difficult to change, worth keeping or ready to be altered or ignored given the purposes at hand. The former way of thinking is in keeping with concern about control of bureaucracy, and the latter fits the pragmatic emphasis on a future formed in the process of discourse. John Dewey (1927, p. 65) noted that "to suppose that an *a priori* conception of the intrinsic nature and limits of the individual on one side and the state on the other will yield good results once for all is absurd." Public administrators and citizens who believe it wise to take into account the context of a discourse process need not accept a fixed, reified account of that context.

Within the confines of administrative legitimacy based on control, the range of potential action may be limited by the screening out of information that could threaten elite interests, a predetermined understanding of what is public and what is private, and a definition of the administrator as a neutral expert, despite knowledge that no one is neutral and that clear separation of politics and administration is a fiction. In the perspective of legitimacy based on collaborative discourse, it is acknowledged that existing understandings of the social context and public administration are not fixed certainties that must be preserved, they are the point at which action begins. It is also recognized that contemporary society places actors in a discourse process in a position of challenge and well-chosen opportunity rather than unbridled optimism. It is not always enough to gather people together and assume that they will spontaneously develop a deep understanding of the situation and possibilities. The administrator who chooses to engage in discourse may also need to be an organizer and educator, and success means working toward joint understanding rather than imposing a predetermined agenda on unsuspecting citizens. In this process, administrative legitimacy is created through relationships formed in collaborative interaction, shedding the man-of-reason facade and giving away knowledge and control to citizens. Awareness of the control exerted by institutional and legal constructs is useful to administrators, helping them fulfill organizational and professional obligations. Awareness of the political and economic forces that shape those constructs helps administrators facilitate a discourse process that allows citizens to create the future they desire.

— 6 —

Private Lives
and Antiadministration

Much theory in public administration assumes that citizens are, or should be, deeply involved in public affairs. However, most people are not involved in public discourse, leaving them vulnerable to actions taken by the small percentage of the population who do participate. Public administrators are key actors in shaping perceptions of which problems should rise to the public agenda, what action alternatives are available, and how implementation of programmatic decisions affects members of the public. In this role, they are a remaining buffer between public action and potentially disruptive or damaging impacts on private lives. The paper suggests that in adopting an antiadministrative stance toward administrative action, public professionals might exercise imagination as a means of protecting private lives.

It seems like an odd name for a theory of public administration: "Antiadministration." Also, the content of the theory appears contrary to accepted goals of public administration because it suggests administrators should shed power and control, questioning their own objectives and becoming "tentative" in their commitments. Like the reinvention/new public

From *Administrative Theory & Praxis*, vol. 23 no. 4 (December 2001): 541–558. Copyright © 2001 Public Administration Theory Network. Reprinted with permission.

management/managerialist movement, antiadministration is a response to bureaucracy as a ponderous, rule-bound preserve of program expertise and jargon. However, new public management maximizes technical control and efficiency and, as if in a mirror image, antiadministration would shift determination of public action from managers to citizens.

David John Farmer's antiadministration is part of a small movement in public administration of people desiring to move the field away from a focus on managerial imperatives such as efficiency and control. This is not a matter of abandoning administrative competence, but of being open to multiple views instead of excluding people who disagree with a normative managerial perspective. Antiadministration shares some features with other strands in this movement (Adams et al., 1990; Box, 1998; King & Stivers, 1998; McSwite, 1997), including aversion to bureaucratic control, desire to redistribute knowledge and decision-making capacity, and wariness of large institutional systems. It is based partially on postmodern concepts such as "alterity," an awareness of the moral validity of differing perspectives and the need to avoid stereotyped thinking. Alterity encourages administrators to avoid coercive action that stifles multiple possibilities—to express this thought, Farmer (1995, p. 228) uses a phrase from Michel Foucault, suggesting we tame the "fascism in us all."

Antiadministration is more than citizen involvement by cooptation, consultation, or education. Among other things, antiadministration facilitates "anarchism" (Farmer, 1995, p. 238), seeks "a fundamental redistribution of governmental power in favor of the community" (p. 234), and requires "courageous professionalism" (pp. 243–244) that operates tentatively rather than authoritatively. Farmer asks: "How would corrections agencies tend to behave if they suspected correctional operations and agencies? How would tax managers tend to operate if their moral predisposition was to suspect the institution of taxing and all taxing agencies? How would diplomats tend to behave if they felt a moral imperative against the institution of diplomacy?" (p. 244).

Antiadministration could become rather mundane if summarized in a new set of "proverbs of administration." In place of Gulick's original proverbs, the antiadministration proverbs might ask administrators to treat everyone not as a category but as an individual, to avoid creating policies and programs with a fixed, totalizing vision, and to encourage citizen involvement in governance. At this level, antiadministration would become merely another administrative tool, a different way to think about agency management.

Antiadministration is saved from this fate by offering a perspective in contrast with prevailing models and by our need for it in a time when other ideas do not seem to do what (some think) ought to be done. The history of the democratic impulse is that portions of the citizenry occasionally assert themselves against governmental policy formulated by a small percentage of the people. Public administration often serves as the implementation arm for this small percentage of individuals and groups who exercise influence to shape public action for private benefit. It cannot be assumed these people and groups will behave with awareness of alterity, taking into account the needs of others in addition to their own.

It is argued here that one measure of antiadministration is the extent to which people are able to live private lives without fearing public-sector administrative action that degrades their quality of life. Quality of life may be measured in environmental conditions, good services at low cost, a humane society, or other ends people value or would value if they were aware of the options available to them. In the following sections, the possibilities of such an antiadministration are explored. We begin with a critical, materialist analysis of the society within which antiadministration would operate. Next, a case is made for the importance and value of private lives in addition to the classical republican vision of virtuous citizens. The paper concludes with discussion of the potential for movement toward an antiadministration that protects private lives.

Daily Human Interests

Many human interests related to governmental action are material (they result from the relationship of individuals to economic and political structures in society) and also physically immediate, close by, part of the experienced daily texture of life. Because to some extent the administrative agencies of government reflect the distribution of resources in society, we may expect administrative decisions about material human interests to be significantly influenced by the wealthy and powerful.

We search here for antiadministration not at the abstract level of national or global "policy," but at the level where government most directly interacts with the people it serves. Many of the public services we take for granted today were once considered private functions. Camilla Stivers (2000a, pp. 54–55) writes that in the Progressive era women pushed for solutions to problems of garbage disposal, sanitation, transportation, wages, and hours of work. In many cases, men resisted bringing such matters into the public, governmental sphere for solution, viewing them as private, household things not suited to public discourse and action. In contrast to such supposedly feminine matters, men were interested in the rough affairs of politics and businesslike efficiency. Women, recognizing that the most pressing human interests were those in the immediate environment, advocated for public solutions to "private" problems, engaging in work they called "public motherhood" and "municipal housekeeping" (p. 9). These issues of municipal housekeeping are reflected today in the discourse of community governance. Their concrete impacts can easily be seen both communitywide and in smaller areas such as neighborhoods.

The following subsections argue that government, at least community government, is mostly about matters that are bounded geographically and begin in the daily human interests of neighborhood residents. Discussion over what to do about these matters plays out in a setting of competition for resources within and between neighborhoods and between communities. Overall, community public life is by nature material, concerned with decisions about the distribution of public resources.

Geography

Because of mobility and technology, the idea of place, a specific bounded area, seems to have lost its prominence in defining human association and sense of community. There are now countless thousands of options open to people in connecting with others of similar interests. Though much of human history consists of stories of the relationship between people and place, it is appealing to believe we have moved beyond a primitive connection with geography and are now floating in boundless electronic association, free of the often gritty and disorderly daily neighborhood landscape of people and things that impinge on consciousness and require attention and maintenance.

Today it would be incredibly complex to map individual communication patterns and participation in communities of discussion, business relationships, and so on, even for a relatively small group of people in a small geographic area. For a large, randomly selected sample of people, the research problem would be so complex, with so few overlaps, internal connections, or joint memberships, that it might be argued it no longer makes sense to speak of community as a defined area in which people share joint interests and concerns. This phenomenon is heightened by the rise of individualistic "lifestyle politics," in which "the psychological energy (cathexis) people once devoted to the grand political projects of economic integration and nation-building in industrial democracies is now increasingly directed toward personal projects of managing and expressing complex identities in a fragmenting society. The political attitudes and actions resulting from this emotional work stay much closer to home, and are much less likely to be focused on government" (Bennett, 1998, p. 755).

The desire to break free of geographic determinism and emphasize the possibilities, rather than the limitations, of human self-determination is understandable. If one allows the field of investigation to include whatever interests people have, the picture that emerges is one of individual participation in differentiated layers of association. This complex set of human interrelationships may be described as "multiply-situated selves" (Sandel, 1996, p. 350).

However, if the substantive topic is public administration, then by definition the field of investigation has physical boundaries, since public administration is a function of government and government is defined by boundaries in physical space. The phenomenon of multiply situated selves coexists with the simple fact of geographically defined governmental jurisdictions. If an area is large enough, for example the United States or Europe, we may wish to believe that "community" consists of virtually unlimited options rather than common patterns. But much of the "action" in government today, the innovation, citizen involvement, and the "reforms" of new public management, is local. At this level of government, the connection between people and place becomes particularly evident. People have many interests other than government, but in relation to public action, those who pay attention do so within a geographical framework. Thus, multiply situated selves and geographically centered human interests are not in conflict. Instead, they are based on different units of analysis, the former focusing on individuals and documenting all of their social/associational connections, the latter focusing on public discourse in the governmental sphere, involving only a part of the lives of individuals when it involves them at all.

Neighborhoods

A sample of shared human interests may be found in neighborhoods. At least since Mary Parker Follett's 1918 book *The New State,* we have known that neighborhoods are a focus of citizen activity as people deal with problems generated both from within and from outside the neighborhood. The internet has made it possible to access neighborhood discussions and active sites for electronic sharing of information on local issues. As an example, at the web site for the North Beacon Hill neighborhood in Seattle (as of November 2003, www.ci.seattle.we.us/beaconhill/default1.htm), we find information about planting trees, concerns about conditions in the neighborhood city park, protests against noise from airplanes landing at Seattle-Tacoma airport, photographic tours of the area, a photographic record of a neighborhood summer evening picnic in the park, information on bus routes, the branch library, and meetings of neighborhood groups, histories people have compiled about the area, and more.

It appears that Beacon Hill residents have close working relationships with city staff and the web site has immediate links to the city of Seattle online. Neighborhood residents are sometimes in disagreement with the city when agencies either take action or fail to take action in ways residents believe to be detrimental to the neighborhood. One has the sense from the web site that this is a vibrant, multiethnic neighborhood with many residents who care deeply about it as their home. The area also appears to have problems with maintenance of public properties and some residents think the city is insufficiently attentive to their preferences and needs.

Different neighborhoods face different issues. On web sites for neighborhoods nationwide one may find, for example, emphasis on the impacts of development projects (appearance, traffic, noise, and so on), interest in preservation of neighborhood landmarks, or daily matters such as (from a neighborhood in Eugene, Oregon) loud parties, speeding cars, barking dogs, and alleyways overgrown with weeds. The common theme in these neighborhoods is people banding together to take action on local conditions that may seem mundane compared to the grand scale of national "public policy," but which are significant for daily lives. This common theme connects the physical attributes of neighborhoods with residents' satisfaction with life, because:

> the material use of place cannot he separated from psychological use; the daily round that makes physical survival possible takes on emotional meanings through that very capacity to fulfill life's crucial goals. The material and psychic rewards thus combine to create a feeling of "community." Much of residents' striving as members of community organizations or just as responsible neighbors represents an effort to preserve and enhance their networks of sustenance. Appreciation of neighborhood resources, so varied and diversely experienced, gives rise to "sentiment." Sentiment is the inadequately articulated sense that a particular place uniquely fulfills a complex set of needs. (Logan & Molotch, 1987, p. 20)

Political Economy

The neighborhood is not the only geographic unit important to human interests and governmental action, which can stretch across a city, region, nation, or cross-national area. Superficially, human interests may seem different in the broader world beyond the neighborhood, but all interests dealt with through the collective choice mechanism of government are subject to the limitations of finite public resources. There is competition for these resources and there are winners and losers, since "discrimination cannot be avoided in the allocation of scarce goods" (Johnson, 1991, p. 35).

In such an environment in a community, some seek to use the public, governmental sphere to enhance private interests (this is the public choice economists' "rent-seeking behavior") (pp. 327–340). In communities, those interests are often related to the use of land and buildings, the physical environment that shapes much of the human experience in urban and suburban places. Peterson (1981) described public policy in communities as oriented toward physical and economic development and away from concern with redistributional policies, or what we might call social welfare. This makes the community attractive to businesses looking for a place to locate, thus supposedly providing a benefit for everyone in the community.

Logan & Molotch (1987) argue there are negative impacts to such growth and it enhances "exchange values" (benefits to entrepreneurs from the community as a marketplace) at the expense of "use values" (benefits to residents from the community as a living environment—in the neighborhood, the desire to create and preserve a physical community of safety, esthetic pleasure, and social function). The search to make profits from the community as a marketplace means that competition occurs at several levels simultaneously, in "competitive systems nested within one another" (Logan & Molotch, 1987, p. 35). Thus, "owners of a commercial block compete against owners of the next block, but they unite when their business district competes against other business districts in the same city. The owners of all the business districts in one city stand together in competition with other cities" (p. 35).

In relation to the whole population of the community, those who benefit most from the community as marketplace are a very small percentage. They have the most to gain or lose individually from public actions, such as allocation of tax dollars or environmental regulation, so they have a strong incentive to organize to exert influence on public governing bodies and public administrators. The rest of the people do not have such strong individual incentives to create organized pressure groups (Olson, 1965), and so most of them are not active in public affairs, and may only become so if faced with a specific threat to their immediate environment (the not-in-my-backyard, or NIMBY, syndrome). This gives those with most to gain both the incentive and the opportunity to shape public action to their liking.

The literature of power and governance (Judge, Stoker, & Wolman, 1997; Ricci, 1971; Waste, 1986) indicates that people will use government to achieve personal advantage. Recognition of this tendency may be found in earlier historical periods, for example during the debate about the relationship of government to the individual during the founding of the American nation. Wood (1969) characterizes this debate, in part, as one between socioeconomic classes, as those with less tried to break the monopoly on wealth of those with more. Later expansion of the middle class and the welfare state has smoothed some of the edges off this human drama, but, "insofar as history presents a moral spectacle, it is the struggle to break such monopolies" (Rorty, 1999, p. 206).

Materiality

Returning to the neighborhood for a moment to refocus on daily human interests, we can identify two types of disjunction between the preferences of the individual and the actions of social entities. One is a matter of size, of scale. A good example is concern in the Beacon Hill neighborhood about noise from the regional airport. It would be better for people in the neighborhood if the airport did not exist, but that is not a practical option. It would also be better for people in the neighborhood if airport officials would reallocate air corridors so that fewer planes pass over Beacon Hill. That is discussed in the neighborhood web site; it may or may not be a feasible option from the point of view of airport officials, but it would be a better fit between localized individual concerns and the needs of the larger social entity. In this as in other situations, there is a conflict between human interests on a small scale and on a larger scale. Relationships between units of public discourse may be made smoother and more satisfying by recognizing the importance and value of the small as well as the large. However, even such a "polycentric" acknowledgement of mutual interdependence is subject to "contestation" and the possibility that "some will take advantage of opportunities to gain advantage over others" (Ostrom, 1991, p. 239).

The other type of disjunction between individual preferences and larger social entities is related to the potential clash of use and exchange values, in which "use values of a majority are sacrificed for the exchange gains of the few" (Logan & Molotch, 1987, p. 98). It is simplistic to say that a small class of wealthy entrepreneurs uses the community to make money and everyone else suffers as a result. There are "trickle-down" effects from successful economic competition (Peterson, 1981) and many people who are interested in the community as a living environment also have a stake

116

in its economic health. Their jobs could be threatened by economic weakness, so for economic well-being they are willing to tolerate a certain amount of deterioration in quality of life, for example the esthetic blight of shoddy, cookie-cutter development and highways lined with billboards, decreased air quality, traffic congestion and long commute times, increased crime, poor schools, and insufficient attention to social conditions.

However, some of the tolerated deterioration in quality of life is not necessary for community economic well-being, but is intended to allow surplus transfers of wealth (surplus because they are larger than is necessary to encourage entrepreneurial activity) to those who exercise the greatest control over governmental policies. These people manipulate the public system so the citizenry as a whole pays more than might be thought of as its fair share of the costs of private profit. Examples of situations in which this may occur include having the public rather than developers pay the largest part of costs associated with expansion of streets and water, sewer, and school system capacity associated with a new shopping mall, conference center, manufacturing facility, or sports facility; preventing or minimizing esthetic standards such as regulations that require review of architectural designs or control the size and appearance of signs along streets; preventing public review of proposals for buildings so tall or large they block sunlight and degrade the environment of streets and surrounding buildings; minimizing use of scarce resources in poorer neighborhoods, since people of lower socioeconomic status are less likely to vote than people in wealthier neighborhoods; and preventing or minimizing developer contributions for parks, bicycle/pedestrian paths, and other amenities in new developments; and so on.

In sum, the people with the most to gain from community decisions seek to make money unhindered by the impacts of their actions on others. Public administrators who facilitate this concentration of power and wealth are not value free, but instead make choices every day that affect the nature of democracy (or lack thereof). At the polar extremes of a continuum, the democracy administrators foster may be at one end the sort that favors a certain economic group and set of behaviors, and at the other end one that recognizes a wider range of human interests. There is no simple dichotomy between classes in this story, little evidence of an unchanging, cohesive, easily identifiable elite group, no smoking gun of oppression. There is instead a public governance system that offers rewards to those who play the game a certain way, supplemented by administrative agencies and people who carry out the will of those who "win" the public game.

Avoiding simplistic characterization of the players in this game also means avoiding a stereotypical model of class warfare. It does not, however, mean carrying alterity to the extreme of inability to distinguish desirable outcomes and undesirable outcomes, circumstances that can be accepted and circumstances that need to be changed. For those who view social relationships as material, based on distribution of physical resources and opportunities, a primary concern is to "eliminate the injustices of class differences and the priority of private property and profit" (Ebert, 1996, p. 201).

This sort of injustice is an old story, traceable at least to ancient Athens (Phillips, 1993). In 1787, James Madison wrote that "the most common and durable source of factions has been the various and unequal distribution of property" (in Rossiter, 1961, p. 79). The Levellers of the English revolution in the middle of the seventeenth century reacted against what they saw as oppressive inequalities of wealth and power that deprived people of rights and liberties. One of the more radical egalitarian Levellers, Gerrard Winstanley, "believed that economic freedom must come before personal freedom" (Dow, 1985, p. 75). He asked, "is not buying and selling a righteous law? No, it is the law of the conqueror, and not the righteous law of creation" (quoted in Holorenshaw, 1971, p. 23).

Today, mass capitalist society has been remarkably successful in producing a quantity of physical goods that distracts us from thinking about serious underlying issues. Alterity helps us realize our moral ambivalence and the relativity of opinion and situation. Materiality reminds us that respect and care for others is not the same thing as forsaking critical awareness of circumstances. As Teresa Ebert (1996, p. 201) wrote, "the privileging and mystification of the other is an alibi for placing class interests beyond the reach of change."

Citizenship and Private Lives

We frequently encounter advocacy of a classical republican model of citizenship that portrays engaged and dutiful participants in public discourse who identify their self-worth, at least in part, with their contribution to collective social association (Bang et al., 2000; Barber, 1984). However, this is not reality in most places and for most people. Aside from the problem of citizen mistrust of government, people can be interested in public affairs but not think of themselves as direct participants, or they may pay little attention except when something happens that affects them directly. The pace and content of most people's lives are such that they have little or no time or inclination to function as involved citizens.

O.C. McSwite (1997) has described the extant American governmental system as a product of the Federalist victory in the debate between Federalists and Anti-Federalists over ratification of the Constitution. According to McSwite, this victory enshrined an elite, market-oriented worldview that kept citizens at a distance from control of government because they might threaten stability and economic order. Though this analysis is especially applicable to the national level, the idea that representative government rather than direct democracy is appropriate has affected all levels of government and can be found cross-nationally as well.

Some attention has been given in public administration theory to countering the effects of representative democracy and improving citizen-administrator interaction to facilitate democratic will formation (Box, 1998; Fox & Miller, 1995; King & Stivers, 1998). This is a laudable goal, but because most citizens are not involved in public discourse processes, decisions are often made by self-interested people and by community activists pushing their particular view of the public interest. In 1950s and 1960s research on community power structures conducted by sociologists and political scientists, both elite theorists (who think a cohesive group of people with common interests exercise considerable control over community decision making) and pluralists (who think different people are involved in different issues, so there are many centers of power) concluded that only a small percentage of the population is involved in public affairs (Waste, 1986, p. 17).

What percentage of the general population approaches the classical republican standard of the conscientious citizen who is informed and involved? Some of us who teach the graduate introductory course in public administration notice that many graduate students entering our programs, whether or not they have related work experience, know little about the history, structure, and operation of government at any level, are either not aware of current political, cultural, and economic events that shape society or are aware of them on the level of media sound bites, and are not involved in what we might think of as civic activities. This is a select group of people; by definition, they are interested in public service; many are experienced practitioners, and all have a college degree. If the basics of public life are a surprise to them, we may expect the population as a whole to be largely uninformed and uninvolved.

Some of us have spoken to community leadership training groups including citizens who are already active as community volunteers. These are mostly bright, well-educated people who want to contribute constructively to civic life and expect the speaker to tell them how to make an impact on issues of public governance. Some of them may feel blocked from doing so by lack of understanding of the complexities of public institutions and are intimidated by the legalistic formalism and the highly technical nature of government. They ask, "But how do I start?" and, "Is it really possible for me to make a difference?" If these people have such thoughts, can we expect other citizens to rush into the arena of public discourse, ready to commit dozens of hours to acquiring the knowledge needed to participate fully and successfully?

Behind the idea that an active, involved citizenry is a good thing can be the normative assumption about democracy that governmental action should be shaped by the maximum feasible number of citizens. Another assumption can be that when the public does not actively monitor government, influential people and groups will make decisions contrary to the interests of some or all of the public. The former assumption is counterfactual in relation to actual citizen behavior and the latter assumption places citizens in a defensive posture. If they do not participate continuously (as we seem to think good citizens would) and push to make their preferences part of public decisions, their choices are to monitor public actions and voice concern when something happens of which they disapprove, to accept what others do even if it causes them concern or harm, or to exit by moving to another community (Lowery, De Hoog, & Lyons, 1992).

We need to ask normatively whether it is reasonable, or good, to assume that citizens should be involved in public affairs, either because it is the right way for people to live their lives, or because they must protect themselves from others who are involved. The thread of civic republicanism, the idea that public life is the venue of self-fulfillment, begins with males who were privileged citizens in ancient Athens. In the American setting this thread runs through the desire of the eighteenth-century founding generation for citizens, even in a republic built on recognition of self-interest in the classical liberal style, to exhibit a commitment to "civic virtue." Despite recognizing that "citizens are inclined to be free-riders and rulers are inclined to be tyrants" (Sinopoli, 1992, p. 6), many in this generation hoped to "see civic participation spread over a broad segment of the civic population," to include "activities beyond minimal acts such as voting" (p. 11).

However, in contemporary mass society, maybe it should be acceptable to lead a private life, secure in the knowledge that public services will be provided efficiently and effectively, with few errors and little waste, on a scale and scope appropriate in the sense that most citizens would agree that what is being done is what should be done. This acceptance of private life need not result in subordination of women, minorities, or the poor by putting matters of concern to daily life and the household out of the public sphere (Elshtain, 1981), nor need it be a retreat from society in the manner of Henry David Thoreau's cabin by a pond. Instead, recognizing the social and economic conditions of life, we might stand the classical liberal model on its head. That model uses representative government and bureaucratic expertise (Yankelovich, 1991, calls this particular form of expertise the "Culture of Technical Control") to exclude citizens from governance and protect the interests of the powerful. To accept private lives is to recognize that most people are not involved in the public sphere but should be able, nonetheless, to live lives relatively free from damage set in motion by other citizens and implemented by public administration. This formulation of the citizen-government nexus seeks to bypass the standoff between the classical republican view of participatory citizenship and the pessimistic classical liberal view of control by a self-interested elite. Of course, it may not be any more successful than either model or other attempts at alternative solutions. The point is to try.

Imagination

We have seen that a small percentage of the population is particularly effective in shaping public action for private purposes. Another small percentage of citizens is involved in public governance; their interests may be homogeneous or varied and may or may not be in sympathy with the goals of the first group. Then, last but definitely not least in numbers or significance, the bulk of the population is not directly involved in public governance. Their interests are diverse and may or may not be served by the actions of the first two groups. It is also necessary to recognize the impressive efforts of many people in many places to counter this reality with neighborhood participation groups, citizen boards, and so on (Box, 1998). However, we are dealing here with the aggregate situation rather than the exceptions. To the extent successful efforts toward citizen self-governance can be expanded and spread to other places, this is all to the good, but the topic under discussion is the fate of the bulk of citizens who are either not living in such places or not participating if they do.

Given this setting, there is a clear connection between private lives and antiadministration. If we believe people should he allowed to have private lives free from undue public sector interference, and if elected officials and involved citizens cannot always be expected to serve the interests of the bulk of the people, we are left with public administration as a buffer between citizens and government. This is not to say that public administration is an ideal repository of trust to serve as such a buffer; as noted earlier, it tends to be the instrument of the will of governing elites. It is instead to say, in the framework of antiadministration, that some administrators in some places may seek to adopt an antiadministrative approach, taking the risks associated with countering the dominant sociopolitical paradigm.

For public administrators to intervene to protect private lives, they would need to abandon the ideal of dutiful neutral service and adopt a particular set of values and motivations. Discussion of the problem of what values to assume if public administration is not value neutral has been with the field for some time. It is part of the enduring question of administrative legitimacy, or expressed another way, the politics-administration relationship. The problem of values and neutrality has appeared, for example, in the Friedrich-Finer debate in the 1940s about ethics (McSwite, 1997, pp. 29–52), in Herbert Simon's distinction between fact and value in 1945, and in the 1970s in the emphasis of "new public administration" on the administrator as advocate for social equity. Today, reversing the new public administration model, it appears in new public management as a wish to reassert the politics-administration separation and keep public employees out of policy making.

Rather than move onto this well-trodden path, we may note there are significant barriers to public administrators serving as a buffer between elected representatives and citizens. One barrier is that political leaders may regard this buffer role as a threat, taking defensive actions that could endanger administrators (Box, 1998). Another barrier is that many administrators do not identify their role as being oriented toward citizens, but instead feel allegiance to their profession or to elected or organizational leaders. A third barrier to public administrators serving in a buffer role is the difficulty of identifying citizen interests, because they are often plural, diverse, and conflicting.

The question here is not simply whether administrative action is value laden (how, exactly, could that be avoided anyway?), or whom administrators should serve (elected representatives, citizens, a value or ideal, etc.). Rather, we recognize the diversity of views held by public administrators and instead ask how those who choose to exercise administrative discretion may help in protecting private lives. This requires thinking about the civically uninvolved instead of only about elected representatives, a group of powerful organizations and people, or some involved citizens. It requires an act of empathetic imagination, imagining the daily human interests of citizens and how administrative actions may be tailored to those interests, minimizing the disruptive or damaging effects of public actions.

Public service practitioners have knowledge of practices in vocational specialties (social work, planning, education, law enforcement, and so on) that most citizens do not have. They exercise influence over public actions by making recommendations to decision makers and by deciding how policy is implemented. Practitioners may use their knowledge of practices to shape recommendations to serve what they know of the needs of citizens. If practitioners chose to tailor their recommendations to what they know of private lives, what is it they would know about them? Though private lives cannot be fully imagined, over time practitioners conceptualize patterns of human interests related to the public sphere, built from countless citizen responses to daily matters occurring in thousands of communities. These patterns are revealed to practitioners in the behaviors and speech of citizens who become actively involved in public life, they are revealed in the discourse of citizens who enter the public sphere for only a short time because of an event or issue that troubles them, they are revealed by paying attention to sensory input from daily life, including the media, talk on the street, and the personal living experience of practitioners outside of the professional setting, and they are revealed through education and study.

Not all practitioners are in a position to affect private lives. Of those who are, not all will choose to take into account patterns of revealed human interests, shaping their actions to protect private lives. It is certainly easier to avoid imagining the multiple, complex, dynamic lives that can be affected by administrative action. It is easier not to think about how these lives would be different if public policies and actions were oriented toward unheard citizens instead of the few who have the incentives, knowledge, and time to participate directly in crafting the role of the public sector in the community.

David John Farmer's antiadministration advocates tentativeness, a questioning of administrative systems and actions. This tentativeness fits well with the effort to imagine private lives. It also fits, on a theoretical level, with Chantal Mouffe's (1993, p. 145) vision of a plural/liberal democracy that moves beyond the traditional, natural-law sort of liberal, "rational, universal solution to the problem of political order." Mouffe's democracy is not waiting for "the outcome of a rational choice or a dialogical process of undistorted communication" (p. 145), but instead leaves open questions of what interests are discussed in the public sphere and how to deal with "hegemonic relations," letting them be resolved in public discourse. Thus, democratic society becomes not a goal, but an open-ended dialogue, "a horizon that can never be reached" (p. 146).

A concern may be raised that tentativeness and open-endedness mean an absence of substantive content, of moral purpose, of desire to change things for the better. Mouffe (1993, p. 151) makes the process of democracy, "democratic values and practices," a moral end. Pragmatist Richard Rorty (1999, pp. 260–261) would likely not disagree with this, but he also acknowledges a substantive desire to revive a politics of the left "that centres on the struggle to prevent the rich from ripping off the rest of the country." Rorty calls his view utopian and contrasts it with radicalism. In his interpretation, utopians do not concern themselves with supposed contradictions between superficial appearances and deep "mistakes" being made in the nature of society. Instead, they favor "the contrast between a painful present and a possibly less painful, dimly seen future" (Rorty, 1998a, p. 214). This seems to beg a question about how we would identify a painful situation, that is, lacking a view of what is wrong in society, how would one know to characterize it as painful? Ebert (1996, p. 5) writes that, "utopianism—of any kind—is popular because it disregards existing social contradictions and points to a 'beyond.'"

Administrators may or may not imagine private lives against a (radical) backdrop of perceived discrepancy between the superficial rhetoric of a democratic society and the deeper and often inequitable economic relations that determine the fate of citizens. However, it may not matter whether proposals and actions that could protect private lives are based on a (glass-is-half-empty) conviction that social relations are flawed and oppressive, or on a (glass-is-half-full) desire to improve conditions by acting on behalf of the interests of the uninvolved. Either way, administrators would bring to bear their knowledge of practices to soften the effects of public power on those who cannot, or do not, become involved in determining how that power is used.

To advocate for antiadministrative protection of private lives, we do not need to identify a specific principle (such as democracy in the abstract, or new public administration's social equity, or a more rational or communitarian discourse setting) we think practitioners should pursue. Nor do we need to think naively of this as a panacea, or as anything more than one constructive thing we can do at this lime. We can advocate for it simply because we think, in this supposedly democratic society and at this time, it is the right thing to do. The population of those whose private lives need protection includes people with many different interests and in many different places and times. Each practitioner works from her or his own unique knowledge, experience, and motivation for service. The potential combinations of public issues, practitioner interpretation of imagined private lives, political settings, professional knowledge of practice, and possible substantive outcomes, are virtually infinite. Choices must be made, but beyond imagination, care for private lives, and awareness of the difficulty of knowing for sure what should be done, as theorists we may have neither the need nor the means to ask for more.

— 7 —

Critical Practice and the Problem of Finding a Public

Involving citizens in local governance has long been accepted as a means to improve democracy. However, it is increasingly recognized that most people are not interested in traditional forms of participation in public decision making. This chapter offers an explanatory framework for this phenomenon and a potential response by public practitioners, based on critical social theory. Elements of the framework include contradiction and dialectical change, critical imagination, and self-determination.

Much of the literature of citizen involvement in local governance is based on the idea that more involvement is better than less, because democracy is served by broad participation in self-governance. This "classical republican," or Athenian, model assumes that people want to be involved in decision making on public matters. However, that assumption has been under attack for some time on grounds of empirical inadequacy, since people are not participating in the numbers expected or desired. From the ancient Greeks to the American Federalists and contemporary advocates of representative government, citizen involvement in governance has been resisted because the mass of people are regarded as incapable of understanding public issues and acting rationally. In addition, many professional public administrators believe public involvement in decision making about public services to be inappropriate, either because the public cannot understand how public services work, or because it is inefficient to spend time working with them, or both.

126

There are some bright spots on the map of citizen self-governance, but not all local communities have active citizen self-governance, and in the places that do, often only a relatively small percentage of people participate. Though people continue to care about their local places, a number of factors may limit participation in self-governance, such as competing demands on time, free-rider behavior, lack of knowledge, and aversion to public affairs.

Often, writing about citizen involvement focuses on barriers and techniques. The implicit goal appears to be to create a discourse process that mimics direct democracy to the extent possible: decision making by everyone affected. The purpose of this chapter is not to add to this discussion, but to apply a critical analysis to the matter of describing a "public" capable of self-governing and to suggest elements of a framework for the critical practice of community public administration. By "critical" is meant use of concepts drawn from critical social theory (contradiction and dialectical change; critical imagination; and self-determination) to interpret public affairs at the community level.

The resulting framework for critical practice is intended not as a detailed prescriptive model, but as a means of conceptualizing underlying features of the political and economic system that shape citizen behaviors and constraints on administrative discretion. The framework includes, in the order of sections below, analysis of the problem of locating a self-governing public, description of the challenges facing a critical public practice in local communities, and the purposes of a critical public practice.

The Elusive Public

It has become a cliché in American society that members of the public are indifferent, or even hostile, to government and politics. Voting rates are low, antigovernment attitudes are frequently expressed in the media (talk radio is an extreme example), bureaucrat bashing is commonplace, and the public service is regarded by many with disdain. Elected officials, public professionals, and citizens who are aware of or involved in matters of governance often consider the public to be largely incapable of forming intelligent judgments about public affairs. If public involvement in governing is, or should be, restricted to the periodic act of voting because of apathy or incapacity, then governing is solely the province of elected leaders, their appointees, and public professionals.

The question of whether the public is fit to govern itself is not new. The period of the founding of the Constitutional system was characterized by an intense debate between people in favor of a government that limited public involvement (the Federalists) and people who preferred more direct self-government (Anti-Federalists). Some scholars view the Constitutional period as a reversal of the egalitarian spirit of the Revolution a decade earlier, as those with wealth and power sought to curb what they regarded as an excess of democracy, in the form of greedy, envious, narrow-minded people who threatened their property and status in society. According to Gordon Wood (1969, p. 510), "It was this problem that the federal Constitution was designed to solve." Federalists were pleased to observe that "The scum which was thrown upon the surface by the fermentation of the [Revolutionary] war is daily sinking" (Benjamin Rush, in Wood, 1969, p. 498). The "natural aristocracy" of educated, propertied people hoped to restore their authority over government by shifting the locus of power to the national level, where instead of the people at large taking part in government, it would be controlled by "the purest and noblest characters," who were "the best men in the country" (Wood, 1969, p. 512). Predictably, Anti-Federalists resisted this assertion of power by the "upper" class; Mercy Warren (in Wood, 1969, p. 514) wrote that the Constitution was "a continental exertion of the well-born of America to obtain that darling domination, which they have not been able to accomplish in their respective states"; it "will lead to an aristocratical government, and establish tyranny over us."

Woodrow Wilson's 1887 essay, "The Study of Administration," is studied in public administration especially for Wilson's thoughts on the need to decrease the influence of politics on administration, and for his advocacy of applying "scientific" European management techniques in the American public sector. Often missed are his views about the public. Wilson was writing in the nineteenth century, in which there was a tumultuous democratization of the public sector. In the early years of the century, this democratization was in reaction to the rule of the Federalists at the end of the eighteenth century, then later it was in response to the growth of local government and the changes begun at the national level by presidents such as Thomas Jefferson and Andrew Jackson. Wilson may be viewed as writing against the effects of democratization in the late nineteenth century much as the Federalists sought to curb democracy a century earlier.

On one level, Wilson acknowledged the American expectation that public governance will be the result of democratic policy determined by the people at large. Thus, "administration in the United States must at all points be sensitive to public opinion" (Wilson, [1887] 1997, p. 23). However, Wilson's reasoning placed the public at considerable distance from not only the administration, but also the determination, of public policy. The responsibility for determining the public will belongs to elected representatives and their political appointees, so that "*policy* will have no taint of officialdom about it. It will not be the creation of permanent officials, but of statesmen whose responsibility to public opinion will be direct and inevitable" (p. 23).

This is not an unreasonable thought in a complex, geographically large republic that would be difficult to govern by direct involvement of individual citizens. But because public opinion is characterized by lack of coherence and agreement, Wilson's leaders do not wait for it to form, measuring it to decide what to do next. Instead, they create it: "Whoever would effect a change in a modern constitutional government must first educate his fellow-citizens to want *some* change. That done, he must persuade them to want the particular change he wants. He must first make public opinion willing to listen and then see to it that it listens to the right things. He must stir it up to search for an opinion, and then manage to put the right opinion in its way" (p. 19).

Wilson believed leaders act in this way because the people, individually, are often incapable of rational thought and choice. Instead, they hold "preconceived opinions, *i.e.,* prejudices which are not to be reasoned with because they are not the children of reason" (p. 19). This problem was so severe that even if it were possible for some especially wise people to identify, through study of political history, "a few steady, infallible, placidly wise maxims of government into which all sound political doctrine would be ultimately resolvable" (p. 20), the country might not act on them, because:

> The bulk of mankind is rigidly unphilosophical, and nowadays the bulk of mankind votes. A truth must become not only plain but also commonplace before it will be seen by the people who go to their work very early in the morning; and not to act upon it must involve great and pinching inconveniences before these same people will make up their minds to act upon it.
>
> And where is this unphilosophical bulk of mankind more multifarious in its composition than in the United States? To know the public mind of this country, one must know the mind, not of Americans of the older stocks only, but also of Irishmen, of Germans, of negroes. In order to get a footing for new doctrine, one must influence minds cast in every mould of race, minds inheriting every bias of environment, warped by the histories of a score of different nations, warmed or chilled, closed or expanded by almost every climate of the globe. (p. 20)

This is an image of what today might be called a diverse public, including many people whose conceptions of government and the relationship of individuals to the state may deviate from those held by the educated elite, such as Wilson. In this environment, Wilson considered formation of public opinion and using it to shape administrative implementation to be a problem of how to "make public opinion efficient without suffering it to be meddlesome," since, "directly exercised, in the oversight of the daily details and in the choice of the daily means of government, public criticism is of course a clumsy nuisance, a rustic handling delicate machinery" (p. 23).

In the early twentieth century, Walter Lippmann wrote *Public Opinion* (1922) and *The Phantom Public* (1927), arguing that the world of public affairs was too complex for the ordinary citizen to comprehend. As a result, most people were not directly involved in public decision making, but instead made periodic ballot choices for candidates based on limited knowledge and stereotypes. Since only a relatively small number of people were directly involved in shaping public decisions, the traditional model of the "omnicompetent" citizen, fully informed about and engaged in public affairs, did not describe modern conditions.

John Dewey's *The Public and Its Problems* (1927) was in part written to counter Lippmann's gloomy view of the public and democratic decision making. Dewey also found public capacity to govern in need of improvement, noting that "the prime condition of a democratically organized public is a kind of knowledge and insight which does not yet exist" (p. 166). Instead, "what is applied and employed as the alternative to knowledge in regulation of society is ignorance, prejudice, class-interest and accident," and science and knowledge are used "for pecuniary ends to the profit of a few" (p. 174). This is achieved by influencing public opinion. In a passage that seems quite contemporary in our age of global electronic communication and media consolidation, Dewey wrote that:

> The smoothest road to control of political conduct is by control of opinion. As long as interests of pecuniary profit are powerful, and a public has not located and identified itself, those who have this interest will have an unresisted motive for tampering with the springs of political action in all that affects them. . . . Just as industry conducted by engineers on a factual technical basis would be a very different thing from what it actually is, so the assembling and reporting of news would be a very different thing if the genuine interests of reporters were permitted to work freely. (p. 182)

Observing the growth of the modern administrative state, Dewey worried that "no government by experts in which the masses do not have the chance to inform the experts as to their needs can be anything but an oligarchy managed in the interests of the few" (p. 208). His proposed solution to this situation fit the progressive community-building spirit of the times and bears resemblance to concepts in Mary Parker Follett's *The New State: Group Organization the Solution of Popular Government,* published in 1918. It would require a focus on open discourse, beginning in the "neighborly community" and involving "improvement of the methods and conditions of debate, discussion and persuasion" (Dewey, 1927, p. 208). However, there is much to be done before this "problem of the public" can be solved: "Until secrecy, prejudice, bias, misrepresentation, and propaganda as well as sheer ignorance are replaced by inquiry and publicity, we have no way of telling how apt for judgment of social policies the existing intelligence of the masses may be" (p. 209).

It may be argued that, contrary to Dewey's hopes, the public grows more distant from the process of public governance as society and government become larger and more complex. Steven Best and Douglas Kellner (1997) trace writing on the relationship of the media and public opinion from Danish philosopher Søren Kierkegaard in the mid-nineteenth century, through the "Situationists'" concept of "spectacle" and Jean Baudrillard's postmodern "hyperreality" in the mid- to late twentieth century. One may extract from these materials the idea that people are passive and conformist in the midst of a flood of images that "stupefies social subjects" (p. 84). It redirects public anger from "exploitation and injustice" so that people are "mollified by new cultural productions, social services, and wage increases," and society becomes "a means of advancing profit and gaining ideological control over individuals" (p. 85). In the work of Baudrillard, even the reality behind the image vanishes, leaving only self-referring simulation and little possibility of social resistance. Best and Kellner reject this "nihilistic acceptance of the triumph of the object," preferring to think of contemporary society as "an *intensification* of (capitalist) modernity rather than as a wholly 'new' postmodernity," which is "best understood as a generalized extension of capitalism" (p. 105).

In continuation of the patterns identified by earlier authors, contemporary mass public opinion appears to follow simplistic and sensationalist television and radio programs and the public pronouncements of politicians using the rhetoric of nationalism or public interest to promote the interests of particular groups or businesses. Theorists of participative or deliberative democracy (Barber, 1984; Bohman, 1996; Fung & Wright, 2003; Yankelovich, 1991) and communitarianism (Etzioni, 1998; Sandel, 1996) seek to build public capacity to govern by providing information and engaging groups of people in public discussion, but these efforts affect a small percentage of citizens and likely will not significantly alter overall trends. A citizen involvement and neighborhood organization revival has been occurring at the local level (Berry, Portney, & Thomson, 1993; Box, 1998; Musso, 1999), but it too affects a relatively small percentage of the total national population.

Meanwhile, there is evidence that individual engagement in public issues continues, but its focus has changed from long-term interest in political parties and stable collective identity, to personal identity expressed through changing involvement with multiple issues, campaigns, fundraising appeals, and volunteer efforts (Bennett, 1998). According to Bennett, "sustained levels of volunteer activity further support a story about continuing, but lifestyle-friendly, civic engagement on the part of increasingly individualistic people leading complex lives." People who participate in these new forms of engagement may be among the citizens who "seem to have reached the conclusion that governments are, at worst, responsible for the economic conditions that dominate private lives, and, at best, of little use for remedying them" (1998, p. 758).

There is a theme running through the outline above of the problem of finding a public capable of self-governing. It is the relationship between the public and a governance system dominated by those with wealth and power. It has become fashionable in "postmodern" times to discount theory itself as metanarrative, and comprehensive theories of society involving inequalities in wealth and power as inappropriate claims to a particular truth. Theories based on economic materialism and the work of Marx are particularly antithetical to postmodern thought (Rosenau, 1992, pp. 157–164) and images of the inevitable revolution of the proletariat have faded from the writing of people interested in social justice. However, not only have the effects of capitalism on people and the physical environment remained the central problem of society, they have intensified with growth, globalization, and technological innovation. Frankfurt school critical theorist Herbert Marcuse was deeply involved in adapting concepts that many people think outdated to the task of understanding contemporary conditions (Kellner, 1984, p. 453). Today, this project is more important than ever (Agger, 2002).

For the purpose of this essay—describing a framework for critical practice—it is helpful to assume a model of the political and economic surroundings of public knowledge and action and the contribution of public service practitioners. A particularly useful model is Marcuse's "one-dimensionality." Building on the work of Karl Marx and Max Weber, Marcuse recognized that "domination has its origins . . . in the organization of labor and technology" (Kellner, 1984, p. 166). The instrumental rationality of capitalism is used to extract labor from the public and keep them in a condition of dependence and submissiveness. Box (2003, p. 47) summarized this perspective as follows:

> Contemporary workers are integrated into a system of production and consumption that demands their full commitment to performing the often routine and boring tasks required to make a living. There is a "progressing transfer of power from the human individual to the technical or bureaucratic apparatus" (Marcuse, 2001b, p. 65), and the system rewards conformity and compliance with material goods. Institutions of media, entertainment, education, and politics reinforce the message that production and consumption is good and the resulting environmental degradation is acceptable.
>
> In this situation, the political and economic system swallows up knowledge of alternatives, as "the world tends to become the stuff of total administration, which absorbs even the administrators" (Marcuse, 1964, p. 169). The essential characteristic of such a world is that society, people, and thought are *one-dimensional* (Kellner, 1984, pp. 234–235); that is, knowledge of contradictions has become vague or non-existent and dialectic as an engine of social change has ceased to function.

The search for a specific class of people to overthrow the existing order proved futile in the face of modern urban-industrial society, which provides life-sustaining basics to most and a comfortable life to many. The likelihood of seeking, and finding, better alternatives to the current societal situation diminished as well, as the phenomenon of one-dimensionality resulted in a "flattening out of the contrast (or conflict) between the given and the possible, between the satisfied and the unsatisfied needs" (Marcuse, 1964, p. 8). It became nearly impossible to envision political, economic, or social circumstances different from those to which people have become accustomed, alterity. In this setting the idea of "free and equal discussion" is largely meaningless, because people do not have available the knowledge that would allow "expression and development of independent thinking, free from indoctrination, manipulation, extraneous authority" (Marcuse, 1965, p. 93). Instead, "Under the rule of monopolistic media—themselves the mere instruments of economic and political power—a mentality is created for which right and wrong, true and false are predefined wherever they affect the vital interests of the society" (p. 95). Thus, people become "manipulated and indoctrinated individuals who parrot, as their own, the opinion of their masters" (p. 90). These circumstances certainly make it challenging to locate a public willing and capable of organizing and participating in creating social change, as well as public service practitioners to serve as facilitators of change.

Critical Theory and the Community Context

Turning from discussion of macro characteristics of society to the local community, the possibility that community residents might play a significant role in governance depends on contextual factors such as the public issues currently drawing attention, the socioeconomic characteristics of residents, and the degree to which information and the public decision-making process are open to residents or restricted by community elites. These factors make it more or less difficult for people to bring challenging or controversial issues to public attention.

There are a number of conceptual frames that could be used to describe the political and economic settings in which people become aware of public issues, connect with others to discuss them, and interact with agencies and elected officials to participate in decision making. The frame discussed here is critical theory, which is not a single body of thought with standardized characteristics, but an approach to societal analysis taken by a number of authors. Critical theory focuses on the impacts of the economic system, in particular relationships of wealth and power, with the hope that people can become aware of their circumstances and take action to improve them. It is difficult to generalize about the work of critical theorists because there are significant differences within this category of theory. The Frankfurt school developed a social critique that continues to influence interpretation of society, whether through application to current social problems or in the opposition of those (including Marxists) who disagree with it or think it out of date, "dead" (Bottomore, 2002, p. 76).

Focusing on the work of Marcuse, three ideas may be used as a process framework to address the problem of local self-governance: dialectical change, critical imagination, and self-determination. Dialectical change is the idea that over time current conditions will become qualitatively different. Present "realities" we think of as inevitable or "given" are instead inherently "self-contradictory, opposed to themselves" (Marcuse, 1941, p. 147), and thus subject to transformation. As a result, "social change is no longer a particular event within a rather static reality, but the primary reality itself from which all static [conditions] must be explained" (Marcuse & Neumann, [ca. 1941–42] 1998, p. 102).

The term "critical imagination" is a construction from Marcuse's writing about the use of fantasy, imagination, to envision possible alternative future conditions and actions that might be taken to facilitate change. In this form, it is a means of bridging the "abyss" between a desired future and present reality (Marcuse, 1968, p. 154). Self-determination is the idea that humans seek to make life choices free from coercion. It may be expressed as freedom, liberty, empowerment, and so on, but whatever the specific form the idea is central to critical theory (and is common in the broader field of political theory).

This process framework of dialectical change, critical imagination, and self-determination may be applied to public service and to local governance. In public service, a central contradiction is the difference between the idea that government is formed to act in the interests of the public generally, and the perception that instead it is used to benefit those who exert the most power by use of force, wealth, manipulation of information and the public decision agenda, or other forms of coercion or influence.

Though a variety of issues arise in local governments, a primary motivating factor in local politics and creation of public policy is control over the use of land and buildings to generate profit and accumulate wealth (Logan & Molotch, 1987; Peterson, 1981). The contradiction between acting in the interests of the public and acting for the benefit of those who exert the most power is particularly apparent in the local geography of profit. Geographer David Harvey (2001, p. 83) acknowledges that to mainstream social scientists, focusing on the accumulation of wealth related to land use "probably sounds very economistic and reductionist," and research into urban life involves "much more than the 'mere' study of the physical artifact that is the city." Nevertheless, according to Harvey:

> The whole thrust of the Marxian argument is, of course, to concentrate on the social meaning of things. Starting with the physical artifact that is the city, we can reach out, step by step, into the myriad social relations (between landlords and financiers, building laborers, artisans and capitalist builders, between users and producers, between the state and individuals, between communities and speculators, and so on) and into the extraordinary complexity of interactions, conflicts, coalitions within a framework of institutional arrangements, all of which lead to the creation of this physical landscape. (p. 83)

Thus we find that many elements of the urban environment affecting the daily lives of millions are determined, in large part for their own benefit, by people motivated to use that environment to accumulate wealth. In the words of John Logan and Harvey Molotch (1987, p. 12), "people dreaming, planning, and organizing themselves to make money from property are the agents through which accumulation does its work at the level of the urban place." The affected elements of the urban environment range from the macro scale and well known (proliferation of freeways; urban sprawl; inadequate public transportation; air, water, and noise pollution;

problems with water supply, sewage and waste disposal; and so on), to smaller-scale matters that affect people on a daily basis whether they know it or not, influencing, for example, visual appearance of the urban area, time spent in travel, levels of danger and risk, and satisfaction or frustration with the quality and responsiveness of governmental services.

To use an example from the category of smaller-scale matters, most people are not aware of the practices associated with design of commercial streetscapes. This sounds like a trivial matter, but is in fact a complex area of practice developed over several decades that can have significant impacts on driving safety, the visual environment, the attractiveness of businesses, and possibly the mental image of the community held by residents and outsiders. Envision a typical commercial roadway strip with above-ground utility lines, lots of pavement, large, tall, garish, and often poorly maintained signs, and unlimited driveway access cuts in the curbs (thus unlimited vehicle turning movements on and off the highway). Then, visualize the same strip with the same businesses, except now the utility lines are underground, there are street trees and areas of landscaping, the signs are lower to the ground, of modest size and design and well maintained, and access is limited to a few driveways shared by several businesses each. Driving is safer, the effect of the visual environment on the passer-by or business customer is much different, and public perception of the businesses, and the community overall, may be improved. These objectives can be achieved by adopting well-known and readily available regulatory planning techniques.

However, business owners often resist more attractive street design, sometimes on the basis of cost (though many elements of improved street design are not particularly expensive and some costs may be borne by funding arrangements that reduce costs to businesses), and often because they want to avoid additional regulation that might force them to conform to design norms imposed by the community. People may insist on their "right" to compete by, for example, paving every square foot of property available rather than including some landscaping, creating several access points from the street instead of providing one or two access points, and installing the tallest, largest, multicolored flashing electrical sign they can afford.

This attitude seems to be an artifact of the underlying value of individualism that is deeply entrenched in liberal-capitalist market society, especially in the United States. It is not unique to property or business owners and is not a matter of normatively incorrect belief or unusually self-interested behavior. Rather, it is a matter of responding to proposed change from within a particular understanding about the relationship of the individual to the collectivity, an understanding based on historical knowledge of practices and accepted values. Within this understanding, it is reasonable to expect people to resist public action that would force change in current or future streetscapes, preserving their preference for an individualistic community as contrasted with one in which people plan their living space together.

This resistance may take the form of discussing the matter with appointed planning commissioners and elected city council members, hiring attorneys or private-sector planners to oppose proposals or actions of the public planning staff, encouraging elected officials or senior administrators to silence or fire planners who suggest measures of which they do not approve, and so on. It is often the case that appointed or elected local leaders are themselves involved in making money from property and will support a position against public discussion of alternatives and potential change in policy. In some places, opposition to the individualist/market orientation and in favor of identification of a community public interest becomes evident on commissions and councils, allowing planners greater freedom to introduce possibilities for change (Box, 1998).

Attempts by professional planners to make available to the public information about regulatory techniques for changing streetscapes may be regarded as a direct, insubordinate threat to the authority of elected officials. Most people are unaware that design of streetscapes affecting the daily lives of residents can be consciously chosen by the public and are not necessarily the random result of individual actions. If made aware of available planning techniques, some residents might identify their interests with those of business owners and elected leaders, since market individualism is pervasive in the culture, but some might wish to discuss alternatives or support others who wish to do so. If a discussion ensues it may be heated, with opponents of change, for example, characterizing professional planners as outsiders with a collectivistic agenda. It is common for planners and other public professionals to be fired for initiating discussion of change or for implementing new regulations when change has been made. As Charles Hoch (1994, pp. 1–2) notes, "Professional planners face a serious problem in our liberal democratic society. . . . Planners inhabit a precarious institutional and professional position in the United States, stemming from the tension between individual purposes and the common good and between professional judgment and citizen preferences."

These citizen preferences, because of apathy, lack of information, manipulation of information through public relations programs and suppression of discussion of controversial issues, indoctrination by the elite (for example through "leadership" training programs), and the effects of the one-dimensional society that obscures knowledge of alternatives, may bear little resemblance to public preferences in a setting with open access to information and decision making, that is, in a setting of self-determination. Nevertheless, the distinction between the interests of the general public and the political and economic elite that structures and uses the public sector for its own benefit should not be overdrawn.

Logan and Molotch (1987) adapt the Marxian categories of "exchange value" and "use value" to make this distinction. Exchange value is the economic value of the urban environment as a place to make money and "use value" is the esthetic value of the urban environment as a place to live. This is a useful distinction, but even a public fully informed and empowered to change community practices may not choose to pursue use values alone. Paul Peterson (1981) made the economic argument that everyone is in the same economic boat in a local area, and that the success of people with wealth will benefit those lower on the socioeconomic scale. Though this "trickle-down" model has been used by neoconservatives to justify redistributive policies that benefit the rich at the expense of the majority of people, it is also true that many people have a stake in the economic well-being of a community. Granted there are trade-offs between growth and its effects, for example air pollution and traffic congestion, most people would not welcome economic stagnation or contraction that could threaten their jobs. If the use of wealth and power to restrict public knowledge and access to the decision-making process is not a clear-cut matter of a small elite dominating the masses, it becomes a nuanced situation involving how information is made available and how open and welcoming the decision-making process is to involvement by those who choose to take part.

In the critical theory framework of change, critical imagination, and self-determination, there is a potential contradiction between the interests of the public and the interests of those with most influence over the actions of government. The presence of such contradiction cannot be known unless the public has full information and opportunity to participate in the decision-making process; even then, with conceptual preconditioning in the one-dimensional society, it may be difficult to be certain. However, there may be a number of situations in which the contradiction is relatively clear and a significant portion of residents prefer to examine alternatives to the status quo, making change a possibility. In these situations, critical imagination can be engaged to envision different community futures.

Envisioning different community futures assumes the possibility of citizen intervention in a public policy process controlled by the economic elite. For some community residents, in particular contexts, this possibility may not exist. Using a case example of urban redevelopment, Scott Cummings and Edmond Snider found that the powerful use the tools of land-use regulation to move poor people wherever it will be to their greatest benefit. As they put it, "strategic code enforcement activities in American cities are best understood as a manifestation of class conflict over land use within an urban area" (1988, p. 156). Thus, as the better off seek improvement in residential location, "the poor and working classes are simply moved or displaced to another geographic area of the city, like pawns on a rich man's chess board" (p. 178).

Another example commonly encountered is the use of fees associated with construction permits to offset the cost of expansion of systems such as sewage collection and treatment, treatment and delivery of water, construction of parks and schools, expansion of major streets, and so on. Charging such fees shifts costs of future system expansion necessitated by growth from current residents and business owners to developers or purchasers of new homes or commercial buildings (Logan & Molotch, 1987, pp. 86–88; Nelson, 2000, pp. 391, 412–413). However, developers and others who profit from development (landowners, realtors, attorneys, bankers, suppliers of building materials, and so on) may pressure elected officials and professional staff to keep systems fees low, avoiding public comparisons of fee levels with other communities and analysis of the actual cost of future system expansion on current residents. If such information becomes public despite efforts to suppress it, the supply-side argument may be made that investment in growth is of benefit to all, since with population growth comes increased economic opportunity. Discussion of costs related to congestion, pollution, and demand for increased capacity of streets, schools, and other public infrastructure is avoided unless raised by citizens concerned about growth.

There are, despite these examples of manipulation of public knowledge, opportunities for self-governance. Returning to the streetscape example, if informed community residents recognize a contradiction between current practices and what they wish for their common future, imagine what might be, and take action to influence public regulatory actions, they have begun the process of self-determination. Over time, this may result in a community with a significantly different appearance as well as a more open and democratic governance. This probably does not mean that community affairs will always be peaceful or consensual. As Chantal Mouffe (2000, p. 104) writes, "a well-functioning democracy calls for a vibrant clash of democratic political positions," characteristic of "the dimension of undecidability and the ineradicability of antagonism which are constitutive of the political" (p. 105).

The Purpose of Critical Practice

The discussion above outlines historical and contemporary challenges in locating a self-governing public and uses a critical perspective to describe the community political and economic context. It suggests that the historical tension between social control by the wealthy and powerful and the needs of the mass of citizens has resolved, in contemporary global capitalism, into a setting in which knowledge of alternatives becomes faint or nonexistent and relatively few people wish to participate in public sector governance. This "one-dimensionality" can be found in local communities, where, though the possibilities for self-governance are often not especially promising, there remains potential for enacting alternative futures. There are thousands of local communities, so there is significant variation in the potential for change. In some places the community elite will be progressive in recognizing a civic duty to share opportunities, but in many other places use of public power to secure personal benefit will characterize the pattern of public decision making. In some places citizens will insist on access to the public decision-making process, and in other places they will, to a greater or lesser degree, be passive.

An enduring question in public administration is how much public service practitioners can, and should, legitimately do to change current equilibria in knowledge and power, and how change can be effected within the extant legal and political system. Not all practitioners recognize contradiction and wish to initiate change. Some accept one-dimensional thinking and are fully integrated into the status quo, and some think of themselves as neutral functionaries whatever the nature of the surrounding political and economic system, ready to receive policy direction from above within the representative system of "overhead democracy." There are also models of the roles of public service professionals involving exercise of administrative discretion (Wamsley et al., 1990), and social change informed by critical theory (Box, 1995, 1998; Zanetti, 1997).

However, in today's political and economic environment, the role of the public practitioner as entrepreneurial market manager is dominant, as political leaders push to "run government like a business." The objective here is not to reopen or extend discussion of roles for public service practitioners, but instead to describe a political and economic framework for understanding critical practice at the community level. This framework may be used by practitioners who wish to create openings and opportunities for people, however small a portion of the population, to become knowledgeable about options for the future and methods of enacting them.

Critical theory has had limited discussion and application in public administration. This could be because in one-dimensional society people have become unaware of potential alternatives, or they do not want to see contradictions because it could be upsetting or dangerous to challenge the status quo, or the sort of social problems that inspire critical thought have been resolved, eliminating the need to consider futures different in values and purposes from the present. Justifications for accepting the given and erasing knowledge of alternatives may be found in the narratives of postmodernism, neoconservatism, and consumerism; in each the dialectic of change has receded into vague memory. Calls for critical theory in public administration have diminished in the past two decades, replaced by the metaphor of the market to the extent that conceptualization of possibilities beyond efficient technicism seems wistful, nostalgic, and foolishly utopian. Although before it seemed possible, if not likely, that people might choose to change the course of events as they began to do in the 1960s and 1970s (the women's movement, civil rights, the environment), now it seems all one can hope for is to minimize regression toward earlier societal understandings of people, government, and the physical environment. As defined by Ben Agger (2002, p. 205), this regression is "an undoing of the modernist project in the direction not of a world-weary, post-political postmodernism but of barbarism, Luddism, and the rejection of science."

It is not difficult to argue that problems that would inspire critical thought have not been resolved and that critical theory is needed now more than ever. Below are extracts from a description of contemporary society by Best and Kellner (2001):

> In the United States, the "New Deal" of the 1930s and the "Great Society" of the 1960s have devolved into a dysfunctional welfare state, which in the 1990s produced a disciplinary workfare camp and prison-industrial complex, while millions continued to fall through tears in the "social safety net." Around the globe, neoliberalism has replaced social democracy. With the collapse of the Soviet Union, a predatory global capitalism and its hyper-commodified McCulture are now hegemonic, confronted with no alternative historical bloc. (p. 2)
>
> . . . The past decade of highly uneven economic development has seen escalating urban violence, a wave of teen murders, the proliferation of guns, intensifying hate crimes, a high level of drug and alcohol addiction, steadily increasing divorce rates, declining wages for many, unprecedented levels of

consumer debt, and growing divisions between the haves and the have nots. In this grave new high-tech world, existence is becoming stranger and increasingly dangerous. (p. 3)

This gloomy image could be extended with discussion of the effects of economic expansion on the environment, unilateral military invasions, terrorist attacks, famine, civil wars, the AIDS epidemic in Africa, and so on. The effects of these conditions are felt not just at the level of the nation-state, but everywhere, down to the smallest community. This reflects intensification of individualist liberal-capitalism and the imperatives of technology, organizations, and work narrated by Marcuse. This is indeed a one-dimensional reality in which the level of social control required to preserve civilization has been dramatically surpassed, producing what Marcuse (1955, pp. 21–54) labeled "surplus repression." A one-dimensional, repressive reality supports contemporary political and economic institutions, which constitute "an acquisitive and antagonistic society in the process of constant expansion" (p. 45), producing control and domination within workplaces and in private lives. This setting has been recognized in public administration, though not broadly (Adams et al., 1990; Box et al., 2001).

At its extreme, critical theory can find social conditions under fascism, capitalism, or state socialism so inhumane and alienating that no escape is imaginable. Possible action by those favoring social change would be limited to an all-or-nothing dream of utopian society, a renunciation of any change if it cannot be complete. Frankfurt school theorists Horkheimer and Adorno found themselves in this conceptual situation because their perception of societal conditions was so bleak; the mass media and culture industry had robbed people of even the possibility of imagining alternative futures, so it "appeared that the very existence of contradictions, or at least the consciousness of their existence, was in jeopardy" (Jay, 1973, p. 276).

Marcuse (1972, p. 76) saw in resistance movements of the 1960s and 1970s some hope for social change, though he retained a Marxian commitment to a complete shift from repressive to liberated conditions, rather than partial, incremental reform. He wrote that "reversal of the trend" toward one-dimensional society may begin with "resistance at particular occasions, boycott, non-participation at the local and small group level" (Marcuse, 1965, p. 101).

Since Marcuse's consideration of these matters in the 1970s, it seems that awareness of possibilities for change has narrowed, though Kellner (1989) wrote that the one-dimensional view of society is "deeply flawed." According to Kellner (1989, p. 203, drawing from Marx's account of "Crisis Theory," in *Theories of Surplus Value*), this is because "capitalist societies should be seen as a peculiar combination of streamlined rationality and intense rationality, of organization and disorganization, of crisis tendencies and efforts at crisis management." Periodically, the contradiction between the imperative to produce, consume, and expand to accumulate profit, and the human needs of people for interpersonal connection, fulfillment in work, and a closer relationship to the physical environment comes to the surface, resulting in opportunities for change rather than consistent repression of alternatives.

This is a more optimistic view than that of Marcuse. An argument may be made against it based on changes in global conditions since Kellner wrote almost fifteen years ago, and on a rereading of Marcuse's thought. The changes in global conditions are straightforward; with the collapse of a bipolar world and the increasing dominance of internationalized business, media, and culture (Barber, 1995), it becomes difficult to identify crisis points that create much public awareness of the need for change. Regarding Marcuse's thought, it is easy enough to argue that he was prescient in characterizing politics and the attitudes of the public as increasingly integrated into social and institutional structures. He wrote that "a highly developed consciousness and imagination may generate a vital need for radical change in advanced material conditions. The power of corporate capitalism has stifled the emergence of such a consciousness and imagination; its mass media have adjusted the rational and emotional faculties to its market and its policies and steered them to defense of its dominion" (Marcuse, 1969, p. 15). In this situation, the supposedly democratic political system is instead a means of containing challenges to the extant society, so that "the semi-democratic process works of necessity against radical change because it produces and sustains a popular majority whose opinion is generated by the dominant interests in the *status quo*. As long as this condition prevails, it makes sense to say that the general will is always wrong—wrong inasmuch as it objectively counteracts the possible transformation of society into more humane ways of life" (p. 65).

There is a regressive contemporary shift in the United States toward nationalism, world domination, and reactionary domestic policy designed to enrich a few at the expense of the many and the physical environment. It is supported by a created public opinion that is often ignorant and simplistic, favoring coercive and punitive solutions to public problems. One may argue such circumstances are not new, pointing for example to the McCarthy era of the 1950s or attitudes during the Vietnam War. However accurate this may be, the question now is whether there is a possibility of this powerful combination of forces weakening and presenting openings for alternative thought and action. The 1950s gave way to the 1960s, but from the

1980s through the early years of the new century, society appears to be moving only in the direction described by Marcuse.

Best and Kellner (1991) advocate a "reconstruction of critical social theory" in "techno-capitalist" society. In agreement with postmodern theory, a reconstructed critical theory would recognize the plurality and difference present in the contemporary setting, but it would not hesitate to theorize that setting, because: "Yet against Lyotard and others who reject macrotheory, systemic analysis, or grand historical narratives, we would argue that precisely now we need such comprehensive theories to attempt to capture the new totalizations being undertaken by capitalism in the realm of consumption, the media, information, and so on. From this perspective, one needs new critical theories to conceptualize, describe and interpret macro social processes" (p. 301). The postmodern aversion to "systemic and historical theory" is, for Best and Kellner, "problematical" (p. 273), because without it, "we are condemned to live among the fragments without clear indications of what impact new technologies and social developments are having on the various domains of our social life" (p. 301).

Though the framework for a critical practice suggested here (dialectical change; critical imagination; self-determination) draws upon a somewhat different analysis of social conditions and set of theories from Best and Kellner's proposed reconstruction, the purpose is the same. It is the application of critical concepts to aid in development of social theory and practice, making possible movement toward alternatives to the given reality. It is not argued that this framework should be primary for all theorists and practitioners, competing to displace all other models. Instead, some may find it useful as a primary conceptual tool and for others it may serve as backdrop to models of the daily practice of professional tasks, such as the critical models of the "participatory researcher" (Zanetti, 1997) or the "helper" (Box, 1998), and models based on social equity, efficiency, legitimacy, discourse, and so on. It also fits well with David John Farmer's (1995) "antiadministration," the idea that public practitioners should exercise their powers carefully, tentatively, and with care for "private lives" (Box, 2001).

A critical framework assumes the characteristics of advanced industrial (or early postmodern; the reader's choice) society described above. Thus, the economic imperative of production, consumption, and accumulation is a significant feature of the social context, with recognition of related features of society in the areas of the media and civil society as well as the presence of localized points of resistance in literature, the arts, and in protests against globalization, restrictions on personal liberties, damaging development, and so on.

In some circumstances, particular public service practitioners may find it desirable to encourage social change through a process of identifying contradictions, imagining the possibilities for change, and assisting people in discovering means of self-determination. In part, they may do this by providing knowledge about historical practices, possible alternatives to current practices, legal and institutional constraints and techniques for changing them, the political and economic context, and the relationship between the public interest (however complex, plural, and fluid the concept may be) and current conditions.

In addition to providing knowledge, practitioners may also make available access to the decision-making process in the form of arranging and facilitating meetings (discourse settings), bringing citizens together with professional and political decision makers, and advising on matters of process and substance. These activities may prove to be difficult, complex, or risky, since members of the public will respond in a variety of ways and powerful people who think that citizens with knowledge and access to the decision-making process are dangerous to their interests may move to contain the process and possibly to punish the practitioners involved. Public discourse processes seemingly intended to be participatory and consensual may actually serve to suppress conflictual expression of the impacts of socioeconomic inequality, differential power, and distorted representation of interests (Cohen & Rogers, 2003; Mansbridge, 2003). Fung and Wright (2003) suggest these effects can be offset to some extent by "countervailing power" in the form of local adversarial organizations, but whether this is sufficient, over time and space, to counter the effects of broad societal structures and practices remains to be seen.

Sometimes, working for change may not seem worth the effort and there is indeed cause for pessimism. Harvey (1985, p. 184) describes the plight of urban planners in a political and economic system that thwarts them at every turn: "the planner seems doomed to a life of perpetual frustration," in which "the high-sounding ideals of planning theory are so frequently translated into grubby practices on the ground." However, public professionals who care about constructive social change are likely to retain a sense of hope for the future, despite the difficulty of working within the society described by the critical framework.

References

Adams, G.B., Bowerman, P.V., Dolbeare, K.M., & Stivers, C. (1990). Joining purpose to practice: A democratic identity for the public service. In H.D. Kass & B.L. Catron (Eds.), *Images and identities in public administration* (pp. 219–240). Newbury Park, CA: Sage.

Agger, B. (1992). *The discourse of domination: From the Frankfurt school to postmodernism.* Evanston, IL: Northwestern University Press.

Agger, B. (2002). *Postponing the postmodern: Sociological practices, selves, and theories.* Lanham, MD: Rowman & Littlefield.

Alway, J. (1995). *Critical theory and political possibilities: Conceptions of emancipatory politics in the works of Horkheimer, Adorno, Marcuse, and Habermas.* Westport, CT: Greenwood Press.

Anglin, R. (1990). Diminishing utility: The effect on citizen preferences for local growth. *Urban Affairs Quarterly, 25,* 684–696.

Banfield, E.C., & Wilson, J.Q. (1963). *City politics.* Cambridge, MA: Harvard University Press.

Bang, H.P., Box, R.C., Hansen, A.P., & Neufeld, J.J. (2000). The state and the citizen: Communitarianism in the United States and Denmark. *Administrative Theory & Praxis, 22,* 369–390.

Barber, B.R. (1984). *Strong democracy: Participatory politics for a new age.* Berkeley: University of California Press.

Barber, B.R. (1995). *Jihad vs. McWorld.* New York: Ballantine Books.

Bennett, L.W. (1998). The uncivic culture: Communication, identity, and the rise of lifestyle politics. *Political Science & Politics, 31,* 741–761.

Berkhofer, R.F. (1995). *Beyond the great story: History as text and discourse.* Cambridge, MA: Harvard University Press.

Berry, J.M., Portney, K.E., & Thomson, K. (1993). *The rebirth of urban democracy.* Washington, D.C.: Brookings Institution.

Best, S., & Kellner, D. (1991). *Postmodern theory: Critical interrogations.* New York: Guilford Press.

Best, S., & Kellner, D. (1997). *The postmodern turn.* New York: Guilford Press.

Best, S., & Kellner, D. (2001). *The postmodern adventure: Science, technology, and cultural studies at the third millennium.* New York: Guilford Press.

Betsworth, R.G. (1990). *Social ethics: An examination of American moral traditions.* Louisville, KY: Westminster/John Knox Press.

Bohman, J. (1996). *Public deliberation: Pluralism, complexity, and democracy.* Cambridge, MA: MIT Press.

Booker, M.K. (2001). *Monsters, mushroom clouds, and the Cold War: American science fiction and the roots of postmodernism, 1946–1964.* Westport, CT: Greenwood Press.

Booker, M.K. (2002). *The post-utopian imagination: American culture in the long 1950s.* Westport, CT: Greenwood Press.

Bottomore, T. (1984). *The Frankfurt school and its critics.* London: Routledge.

Bowles, S., & Gintis, H. (1986). *Democracy and capitalism: Property, community, and the contradictions of modern social thought.* New York: Basic Books.

Box, R.C. (1992). The administrator as trustee of the public interest: Normative ideals and daily practice. *Administration and Society, 24,* 323–345.

Box, R.C. (1995). Critical theory and the paradox of discourse. *American Review of Public Administration, 25,* 1–19.

Box, R.C. (1998). *Citizen governance: Leading American communities into the twenty-first century.* Thousand Oaks, CA: Sage Publications.

Box, R.C. (2001). Private lives and anti-administration. *Administrative Theory & Praxis, 23,* 541–558.

Box, R.C. (2002). Pragmatic discourse and administrative legitimacy. *American Review of Public Administration, 32,* 20–39.

Box, R.C. (2003). Contradiction, utopia, and public administration. *Administrative Theory & Praxis, 25,* 243–260.

Box, R.C. (2004). *Public administration and society: Critical issues in American governance.* Armonk, NY: M.E. Sharpe.

Box, R.C., & King, C.S. (2000). The "T"ruth is elsewhere: Critical history. *Administrative Theory & Praxis, 22,* 751–771.

Box, R.C., Marshall, G.S., Reed, B.J., & Reed, C.M. (2001). New public management and substantive democracy. *Public Administration Review, 61,* 608–619.

Braaten, J. (1991). *Habermas's critical theory of society.* Albany: State University of New York Press.

Burrell, G., & Morgan, G. (1979). *Sociological paradigms and organizational analysis: Elements of the sociology of corporate life.* Portsmouth, NH: Heinemann.

Campbell, J. (1995). *Understanding John Dewey: Nature and cooperative intelligence.* Chicago: Open Court.

Catron, B.L., & Hammond, B.R. (1992). Epilogue: Reflections on practical wisdom—enacting images and developing identity. In H.D. Kass & B.L. Catron (Eds.), *Images and identities in public administration* (pp. 241–251). Newbury Park, CA: Sage.

Cleveland, H. (1985). The twilight of hierarchy: Speculations on the global information society. *Public Administration Review, 45,* 185–195.

Cohen, J., & Rogers, J. (2003). Power and reason. In A. Fung & E.O. Wright (Eds.), *Deepening democracy* (pp. 237–255). London: Verso.

Cooper, T.L. (1991). *An ethic of citizenship for public administration.* Englewood Cliffs, NJ: Prentice Hall.

Cooper, T.L. (1998). *The responsible administrator: An approach to ethics for the administrative role.* San Francisco: Jossey-Bass.

Cornell, S. (1999). *The other founders: Anti-federalism and the dissenting tradition in America, 1788–1828.* Chapel Hill: University of North Carolina Press.

Cummings, S., & Snider, E. (1988). Municipal code enforcement and urban development: Private decisions and public policy in an American city. In S. Cummings (Ed.), *Business elites and urban development: Case studies and critical perspectives* (pp. 153–181). Albany: State University of New York Press.

Dahl, R.A. (1961). *Who governs? Democracy and power in an American city.* New Haven, CT: Yale University Press.

Denhardt, R.B. (1981a). Toward a critical theory of public organization. *Public Administration Review, 41*, 628–635.

Denhardt, R.B. (1981b). *In the shadow of organization.* Lawrence: Regents Press of Kansas.

Dewey, J. (1927). *The public and its problems.* Athens, OH: Swallow Press.

Dow, F.D. (1985). *Radicalism in the English revolution, 1640–1660.* Oxford: Basil Blackwell.

Duby, G. (1985). Ideologies in social history. In J. LeGoff & P. Nora (Eds.), *Constructing the past: Essays in historical methodology* (pp. 151–165). Cambridge, UK: Cambridge University Press.

Dye, T.R., & Zeigler, L.H. (1987). *The irony of democracy: An uncommon introduction to American politics* (7th ed.). Monterey, CA: Brooks/Cole.

Ebert, T.L. (1996). *Ludic feminism and after: Postmodernism, desire, and labor in late capitalism.* Ann Arbor: University of Michigan Press.

Elshtain, J.B. (1981). *Public man, private woman: Women in social and political thought.* Princeton, NJ: Princeton University Press.

Engels, F. (1877). *Anti-Dühring.* Retrieved Oct. 24, 2002, from www.marxists.org/archive/marx/works/1877/anti-duhring/ch10.htm#435, 3.

Etzioni, A. (1998). *The essential communitarian reader.* Lanham, MD: Rowman & Littlefield.

Farmer, D.J. (1995). *The language of public administration: Bureaucracy, modernity, and postmodernity.* Tuscaloosa: University of Alabama Press.

Farmer, D.J. (Ed.). (1998). *Papers on the art of anti-administration.* Burke, VA: Chatelaine Press.

Farmer, D.J. (2000a). Great refusals and the administered life. *Administrative Theory & Praxis, 22,* 640–646.

Farmer, D.J. (2000b). The ladder of organization-think: Beyond flatland. *Administrative Theory & Praxis, 22,* 66–88.

Fay, B. (1987). *Critical social science: Liberation and its limits.* Ithaca, NY: Cornell University Press.

Finer, H. (1941). Administrative responsibility in democratic government. *Public Administration Review, 1,* 335–350.

Follett, M.P. (1998). *The new state: Group organization the solution of popular government.* University Park: Pennsylvania State University Press. (Original work published 1918)

Forester, J. (1980). Critical theory and planning practice. *Journal of the American Planning Association, 46,* 275–286.

Fox, C.J. (1992). What do we mean when we say "professionalism"? A language usage analysis for public administration. *American Review of Public Administration, 22,* 1–17.

Fox, C.J., & Cochran, C.E. (1990). Discretion advocacy in public administration theory: Toward a Platonic guardian class? *Administration and Society, 22,* 249–271.

Fox, C.J., & Miller, H.T. (1995). *Postmodern public administration: Toward discourse.* Thousand Oaks, CA: Sage.

Fraser, N. (1989). *Unruly practices: Power, discourse, and gender in contemporary social theory.* Minneapolis: University of Minnesota Press.

Frazer, F., & Lacey, N. (1993). *The politics of community: A feminist critique of the liberal-communitarian debate.* Toronto: University of Toronto Press.

Frederickson, H.G. (1980). *New public administration.* Tuscaloosa: University of Alabama Press.

Fukuyama, F. (1992). *The end of history and the last man.* New York: Free Press.

Fung, A., & Wright, E.O. (2003). Countervailing power in empowered participatory governance. In A. Fung & E.O. Wright (Eds.), *Deepening democracy: Institutional innovations in empowered participatory governance* (pp. 259–289). London: Verso.

Geuss, R. (1981). *The idea of a critical theory: Habermas and the Frankfurt school.* Cambridge, UK: Cambridge University Press.

Gruber, J.E. (1987). *Controlling bureaucracies: Dilemmas in democratic governance.* Berkeley: University of California Press.

Habermas, J. (1970). *Toward a rational society: Student protest, science, and politics.* Boston: Beacon Press.

Habermas, J. (1998). The different rhythms of philosophy and politics: For Herbert Marcuse on his one hundredth birthday. In D. Kellner (Ed.), *Collected papers of Herbert Marcuse: Towards a critical theory of society* (Vol. 2, pp. 233–238). London: Routledge.

Hansen, K.N. (1998). Identifying facets of democratic administration: The empirical referents of discourse. *Administration & Society, 30,* 443–461.

Harmon, M.M. (1981). *Action theory for public administration.* New York: Longman.

Harrigan, J.J. (1989). *Political change in the metropolis* (4th ed.). Glenview, IL: Scott, Foresman.

Harvey, D. (1985). *The urbanization of capital.* Oxford: Basil Blackwell.

Harvey, D. (2000). *Spaces of hope.* Berkeley: University of California Press.

Harvey, D. (2001). *Spaces of capital: Towards a critical geography.* New York: Routledge.

Hoch, C. (1994). *What planners do: Power, politics and persuasion.* Chicago: Planners Press.

Holorenshaw, H. (1971). *The Levellers and the English revolution.* New York: Howard Fertig.

Horkheimer, M. (1947). *Eclipse of reason.* New York: Continuum.

Horkheimer, M. (1972). *Critical theory: Selected essays.* New York: Herder and Herder.

Horkheimer, M., & Adorno, T. (1944). *Dialectic of enlightenment.* New York: Continuum.

Howe, E., & Kaufman, J. (1979). The ethics of contemporary American planners. *Journal of the American Planning Association, 45,* 243–255.

Hummel, R.P. (1991). Stories managers tell: Why they are valid as science. *Public Administration Review, 51,* 31–41.

Hunter, F. (1953). *Community power structure.* Chapel Hill: University of North Carolina Press.

Jacques, R. (1996). *Manufacturing the employee: Management knowledge from the nineteenth to twenty-first centuries.* Thousand Oaks, CA: Sage.

James, W. (1907). *Pragmatism: A new name for some old ways of thinking.* New York: Longmans, Green.

Jay, M. (1973). *The dialectical imagination: A history of the Frankfurt school and the Institute of Social Research, 1923–1950.* Boston: Little, Brown.

Johnson, D.B. (1991). *Public choice: An introduction to the new political economy.* Mountain View, CA: Mayfield.

Judge, D., Stoker, G., & Wolman, H. (1997). *Theories of urban politics.* Thousand Oaks, CA: Sage.

Kautz, S. (1996). The postmodern self and the politics of liberal education. *Social Philosophy and Policy, 13,* 164–189.

Kellner, D. (1984). *Herbert Marcuse and the crisis of Marxism.* London: Macmillan Education.

Kellner, D. (1989). *Critical theory, Marxism, and modernity.* Baltimore, MD: Johns Hopkins University Press.

Kellner, D. (1998). Preface. In D. Kellner (Ed.), *Technology, war and fascism: Collected papers of Herbert Marcuse* (Vol. 1, pp. xiii–xvi). London: Routledge.

Kellner, D. (2001). Introduction. In D. Kellner (Ed.), *Towards a critical theory of society: Collected papers of Herbert Marcuse* (Vol. 2, pp. 1–33). London: Routledge.

King, C.S. (2000). Talking beyond the rational. *American Review of Public Administration, 30,* 271–291.

King, C.S., & Stivers, C. (1998). *Government is us: Public administration in an anti-government era.* Thousand Oaks, CA: Sage.

Kirlin, J.J. (1996). The big questions of public administration in a democracy. *Public Administration Review, 56,* 416–423.

Kotter, J.P., & Lawrence, P.R. (1974). *Mayors in action: Five approaches to urban governance.* New York: John Wiley and Sons.

Lewis, S. (1991). The town that said no to sprawl. In J.M. DeGrove (Ed.), *Balanced growth: A planning guide for local government* (pp. 18–26). Washington, D.C.: International City Management Association.

Lincoln, Y.S., & Guba, E.G. (1985). *Naturalistic inquiry.* Newbury Park, CA: Sage.

Lippmann, W. (1997). *Public opinion.* New York: Free Press. (Original work published 1922)

Lippmann, W. (2002). *The phantom public.* New Brunswick, NJ: Transaction Publishers. (Original work published 1927)

Logan, J.R., & Molotch, H.L. (1987). *Urban fortunes: The political economy of place.* Berkeley: University of California Press.

Loveridge, R.O. (1971). *City managers in legislative politics.* Indianapolis: Bobbs-Merrill.

Lowery, D., DeHoog, R.H., & Lyons, W.E. (1992). Citizenship in the empowered locality: An elaboration, a critique, and a partial test. *Urban Affairs Quarterly, 28,* 69–103.

Lowi, T.J. (1993). Legitimizing public administration: A disturbed dissent. *Public Administration Review, 53,* 261–264.

Ludtke, A. (Ed.). (1995). *The history of everyday life: Reconstructing historical experiences and ways of life.* Princeton, NJ: Princeton University Press.

Lynd, R.S., & Lynd, H.M. (1937). *Middletown in transition.* New York: Harcourt, Brace.

Lynn, L.E., Jr. (2001). The myth of the bureaucratic paradigm: What traditional public administration really stood for. *Public Administration Review, 61,* 144–160.

Macpherson, C.B. (1977). *The life and times of liberal democracy.* Oxford: Oxford University Press.

Mansbridge, J. (2003). Practice-thought-practice. In A. Fung & E.O. Wright (Eds.), *Deepening democracy* (pp. 175–199). London: Verso.

Marcuse, H. (1941). *Reason and revolution: Hegel and the rise of social theory.* Boston: Beacon Press.

Marcuse, H. (1955). *Eros and civilization: A philosophical inquiry into Freud.* Boston: Beacon Press.

Marcuse, H. (1960). Preface: A note on dialectic. In H. Marcuse, *Reason and revolution: Hegel and the rise of social theory* (pp. vii–xiv). Boston: Beacon Press.

Marcuse, H. (1964). *One-dimensional man: Studies in the ideology of advanced industrial society.* Boston: Beacon Press.

Marcuse, H. (1965). Repressive tolerance. In R.P. Wolff, B. Moore, Jr., & H. Marcuse, *A critique of pure tolerance* (pp. 81–117). Boston: Beacon Press.

Marcuse, H. (1968). *Negations: Essays in critical theory.* Boston: Beacon Press.

Marcuse, H. (1969). *An essay on liberation.* Boston: Beacon Press.

Marcuse, H. (1970). *Five lectures: Psychoanalysis, politics, and utopia.* Boston: Beacon Press.

Marcuse, H. (1972). *Counterrevolution and revolt.* Boston: Beacon Press.

Marcuse, H. (2001a). The problem of social change in the technological society. In D. Kellner (Ed.), *Collected papers of Herbert Marcuse: Towards a critical theory of society* (Vol. 2, pp. 37–57). London: Routledge. (Original work published 1961)

Marcuse, H. (2001b). The individual in the Great Society. In D. Kellner (Ed.), *Collected papers of Herbert Marcuse: Towards a critical theory of society* (Vol. 2, pp. 61–80). London: Routledge. (Original work published 1966)

Marcuse, H. (2001c). Cultural revolution. In D. Kellner (Ed.), *Collected papers of Herbert Marcuse: Towards a critical theory of society* (Vol. 2, pp. 123–162). London: Routledge. (Original work n.d., ca. 1970)

Marcuse, H. (2001d). The historical fate of bourgeois democracy. In D. Kellner (Ed.), *Collected papers of Herbert Marcuse: Towards a critical theory of society* (Vol. 2, pp. 165–186). London: Routledge. (Original work n.d., ca. 1972–73)

Marcuse, H., & Neumann, F. (1998). A history of the doctrine of social change. In D. Kellner (Ed.), *Technology, war, and fascism: Collected papers of Herbert Marcuse* (Vol. 1, pp. 94–104). London: Routledge. (Original work n.d., ca. 1941–42)

Marcuse, H., & Popper, K. (1976). *Revolution or reform? A confrontation.* Chicago: New University Press.

Matthews, R.K. (1984). *The radical politics of Thomas Jefferson: A revisionist view.* Lawrence: University Press of Kansas.

Mattson, K. (1998). *Creating a democratic republic: The struggle for urban participatory democracy during the Progressive era.* University Park: Pennsylvania State University Press.

Mattson, K. (2002). *Intellectuals in action: The origins of the New Left and radical liberalism, 1945–1970.* University Park: Pennsylvania State University Press.

Maurer, R.C., & Christenson, J.A. (1982). Growth and nongrowth orientations of urban, suburban, and rural mayors: Reflections on the city as a growth machine. *Social Science Quarterly, 63,* 350–358.

McDonald, F. (1985). *Novus ordo seclorum: The intellectual origins of the Constitution.* Lawrence: University Press of Kansas.

McSwite, O.C. (1997). *Legitimacy in public administration: A discourse analysis.* Thousand Oaks, CA: Sage.

McSwite, O.C. (1998a). Liberalism (its present and future discontents) and the hope of collaborative pragmatism. *Public Productivity & Management Review, 22,* 271–278.

McSwite, O.C. (1998b). The new normativism and the discourse movement: A meditation. *Administrative Theory & Praxis, 20,* 377–381.

McSwite, O.C. (2000). On the discourse movement—a self interview. *Administrative Theory & Praxis, 22,* 49–65.

McSwite, O.C. (2002). *Invitation to public administration.* Armonk, NY: M.E. Sharpe.

Miller, H.T. (1998). Method: The tail that wants to wag the dog. *Administration & Society, 30,* 462–470.

Miller, H.T., & Nunemaker, J.R. (1999). "Citizen governance" as image management in postmodern context. *Administrative Theory & Praxis, 21,* 302–308.

Mills, C.W. (1958). *The causes of World War Three.* New York: Simon & Schuster.

Mills, C.W. (1959). *The sociological imagination.* London: Oxford University Press.

Mills, C.W. (1962). *The Marxists.* New York: Dell.

Moe, T.M. (1984). The new economics of organization. *American Journal of Political Science, 28,* 739–777.

Molotch, H. (1976). The city as a growth machine: Toward a political economy of place. *American Journal of Sociology, 82,* 309–332.

Mouffe, C. (1993). *The return of the political.* London: Verso.

Mouffe, C. (1996). Deconstruction, pragmatism and the politics of democracy. In C. Mouffe (Ed.), *Deconstruction and pragmatism* (pp. 1–12). London: Routledge.

Mouffe, C. (2000). *The democratic paradox.* London: Verso.

Mumford, L. (1950a). The pragmatic acquiescence. In G. Kennedy (Ed.), *Pragmatism and American culture* (pp. 36–49). Boston: Heath. (Original work published 1926)

Mumford, L. (1950b). The pragmatic acquiescence: A reply. In G. Kennedy (Ed.), *Pragmatism and American culture* (pp. 54–57). Boston: Heath. (Original work published 1927)

Musso, J.A. (1999). Federalism and community in the metropolis: Can Los Angeles neighborhoods help govern Gargantua? *Administrative Theory & Praxis, 21,* 342–353.

Nelson, A.C. (2000). Growth management. In C.J. Hoch, L.C. Dalton, & F.S. So (Eds.), *The practice of local government planning* (3rd ed., pp. 375–399). Washington, D.C.: International City/County Management Association.

Nietzsche, F. (1873). *On the use and abuse of history for life.* Retrieved Dec. 10, 2003 from www.mala.bc.ca/~johnstoi/Nietzsche/history.htm.

Olson, M. (1965). *The logic of collective action: Public goods and the theory of groups.* Cambridge, MA: Harvard University Press.

Ostrom, V. (1991). *The meaning of American federalism.* San Francisco: Institute for Contemporary Studies.

Patterson, P.M. (2000). Nonvirtue is not apathy: Warrants for discourse and citizen dissent. *American Review of Public Administration, 30,* 225–251.

Peterson, P.E. (1981). *City limits.* Chicago: University of Chicago Press.

Phillips, D.L. (1993). *Looking backward: A critical appraisal of communitarian thought.* Princeton, NJ: Princeton University Press.

Putnam, R.D. (2000). *Bowling alone: The collapse and revival of American community.* New York: Simon & Schuster.

Rasmussen, D.M. (1990). *Reading Habermas.* Oxford: Basil Blackwell.

Ricci, D.M. (1971). *Community power and democratic theory: The logic of political analysis.* New York: Random House.

Rohr, J.A. (1978). *Ethics for bureaucrats: An essay on law and values.* New York: Marcel Dekker.

Rohr, J.A. (1986). *To run a constitution: The legitimacy of the administrative state.* Lawrence: University Press of Kansas.

Rohr, J.A. (1993). Toward a more perfect union. *Public Administration Review, 53,* 246–249.

Rorty, R. (1989). *Contingency, irony, and solidarity.* Cambridge, UK: Cambridge University Press.

Rorty, R. (1991). *Objectivity, relativism, and truth.* Cambridge, UK: Cambridge University Press.

Rorty, R. (1996). Response to Simon Critchley. In C. Mouffe (Ed.), *Deconstruction and pragmatism* (pp. 41–46). London: Routledge.

Rorty, R. (1998a). *Truth and progress.* Cambridge, UK: Cambridge University Press.

Rorty, R. (1998b). *Achieving our country: Leftist thought in twentieth-century America.* Cambridge, MA: Harvard University Press.

Rorty, R. (1999). *Philosophy and social hope.* London: Penguin Books.

Rorty, R. (2000). Response to Jürgen Habermas. In R.B. Brandom (Ed.), *Rorty and his critics* (pp. 56–64). Malden, MA: Blackwell.

Rorty, R. (2001). The continuity between the Enlightenment and "postmodernism." In K.M. Baker & P.H. Reill (Eds.), *What's left of Enlightenment? A postmodern question* (pp. 19–36). Stanford, CA: Stanford University Press.

Rosenau, P.M. (1992). *Post-modernism and the social sciences: Insights, inroads, and intrusions.* Princeton, NJ: Princeton University Press.

Ross, B.H., Levine, M.A., & Stedman, M.S., Jr. (1991). *Urban politics: Power in metropolitan America* (4th ed.). Itasca, IL: F.E. Peacock.

Rossiter, R. (Ed.). (1961). *The federalist papers.* New York: New American Library.

Roth, M.S. (1995). *The ironist's cage: Memory, trauma, and the construction of history.* New York: Columbia University Press.

Rousseau, J.J. (1978). *On the social contract, with Geneva manuscript and political economy* (R.D. Masters, Ed.; J.R. Masters, Trans.). New York: St. Martin's Press.

Ruscio, K.P. (1998). Giving reason and politics their due: A response to O.C. McSwite's *Legitimacy in public administration: A discourse analysis. Public Productivity & Management Review, 22,* 268–271.

Ryan, A. (1997). Liberalism. In R.E. Goodin & P. Pettit (Eds.), *A companion to contemporary political philosophy* (pp. 291–311). Oxford: Blackwell.

Ryan, M.P. (1997). *Civic wars: Democracy and public life in the American city during the nineteenth century.* Berkeley: University of California Press.

Sandel, M.J. (1996). *Democracy's discontent: America in search of a public philosophy.* Cambridge, MA: Harvard University Press.

Schattschneider, E.E. (1960). *The semisovereign people: A realist's view of democracy in America.* Hinsdale, IL: Dryden Press.

Schon, D.A. (1971). *Beyond the stable state.* New York: W.W. Norton.

Schon, D.A. (1983). *The reflective practitioner.* New York: Basic Books.

Scott, F.E. (2000). Participative democracy and the transformation of the citizen. *American Review of Public Administration, 30,* 252–270.

Scott, W.G., & Hart, D.K. (1979). *Organizational America.* Boston: Houghton Mifflin.

Sementelli, A.J., & Herzog, R.J. (2000). Framing discourse in budgetary processes: Warrants for normalization and conformity. *Administrative Theory & Praxis, 22,* 105–116.

Sinopoli, R.C. (1992). *The foundations of American citizenship: Liberalism, the Constitution, and civic virtue.* Oxford: Oxford University Press.

Smith, B.G. (1998). *The gender of history: Men, women, and historical practice.* Cambridge, MA: Harvard University Press.

Spicer, M.W., & Terry, L.D. (1993). Legitimacy, history, and logic: Public administration and the Constitution. *Public Administration Review, 53,* 239–246.

Stewart, D.W. (1992). Professionalism vs. democracy: Friedrich vs. Finer revisited. In R.B. Denhardt & B.R. Hammond (Eds.), *Public administration in action: Readings, profiles, and cases* (pp. 156–162). Pacific Grove, CA: Brooks/Cole.

REFERENCES

Stivers, C. (1993). Rationality and romanticism in constitutional argument. *Public Administration Review, 53,* 254–257.

Stivers, C. (1994). The listening bureaucrat: Responsiveness in public administration. *Public Administration Review, 54,* 364–369.

Stivers, C. (2000a). *Bureau men, settlement women: Constructing public administration in the Progressive era.* Lawrence: University Press of Kansas.

Stivers, C. (2000b). Public administration theory as a discourse. *Administrative Theory & Praxis, 22,* 133–139.

Tilman, R. (1984). *C. Wright Mills: A native radical and his American intellectual roots.* University Park: Pennsylvania State University Press.

Tocqueville, Alexis de. (1969). *Democracy in America* (J.P. Mayer, Ed.; G. Lawrence, Trans.). Garden City, NY: Doubleday.

Tucker, R.C. (Ed.). (1972). *The Marx-Engels reader* (2nd ed.). New York: W.W. Norton.

Ventriss, C. (2000). New public management: An examination of its influence on contemporary public affairs and its impact on shaping the intellectual agenda of the field. *Administrative Theory & Praxis, 22,* 500–518.

Vogel, R.K., & Swanson, B.E. (1989). The growth machine versus the antigrowth coalition: The battle for our communities. *Urban Affairs Quarterly, 25,* 63–85.

Waldo, D. (1980). *The enterprise of public administration: A summary view.* Novato, CA: Chandler & Sharp.

Wamsley, G.L., Bacher, R.N., Goodsell, C.T., Kronenberg, P.S., Rohr, J.A., Stivers, C.M., White, O.F., & Wolf, J.A. (1990). *Refounding public administration.* Newbury Park, CA: Sage.

Wamsley, G.L., Goodsell, C.T., Rohr, J.A., Stivers, C.M., White, O.F., & Wolf, J.F. (1987). The public administration and the governance process: Refocusing the American dialogue. In R.C. Chandler (Ed.), *A centennial history of the American administrative state* (pp. 291–317). New York: Free Press.

Warren, K.F. (1993). We have debated ad nauseum the legitimacy of the administrative state—but why? *Public Administration Review, 53,* 249–254.

Waste, R.J. (Ed.). (1986). *Community power: Directions for future research.* Newbury Park, CA: Sage.

Waste, R.J. (1989). *The ecology of city policymaking.* Oxford: Oxford University Press.

White, J.D. (1986). On the growth of knowledge in public administration. *Public Administration Review, 46,* 15–24.

White, J.D. (1990). Images of administrative reason and rationality: The recovery of practical discourse. In H.D. Kass & B.L. Catron (Eds.), *Images and identities in public administration* (pp. 132–150). Newbury Park, CA: Sage.

White, J.D., & Adams, G.B. (1994). Making sense with diversity: The context of research, theory, and knowledge development in public administration. In J.D. White & G.B. Adams, *Research in public administration: Reflections on theory and practice* (pp. 1–24). Thousand Oaks, CA: Sage.

White, O.F., Jr. (1998). The ideology of technocratic empiricism and the discourse movement in contemporary public administration: A clarification. *Administration & Society, 30,* 471–476.

White, O.F., Jr., & McSwain, C.J. (1990). The Phoenix project: Raising a new image of public administration from the ashes of the past. In H.D. Kass & B.L. Catron (Eds.), *Images and identities in public administration* (pp. 21–59). Newbury Park, CA: Sage.

Williams, O.P., & Adrian, C.R. (1963). *Four cities: A study in comparative policy making.* Philadelphia: University of Pennsylvania Press.

Wilson, W. (1997). The study of administration. In J.M. Shafritz & A.C. Hyde (Eds.), *Classics of public administration* (4th ed., pp. 14–26). Fort Worth, TX: Harcourt Brace College Publishers. (Original work published 1887)

Wood, G.S. (1969). *The creation of the American republic 1776–1787.* Chapel Hill: University of North Carolina Press.

Yankelovich, D. (1991). *Coming to public judgment: Making democracy work in a complex world.* Syracuse, NY: Syracuse University Press.

Young, I.M. (2000). *Inclusion and democracy.* Oxford: Oxford University Press.

Zanetti, L.A. (1997). Advancing praxis: Connecting critical theory with practice in public administration. *American Review of Public Administration, 27,* 145–167.

Zanetti, L.A., & Carr, A. (1997). Putting critical theory to work: Giving the public administrator the critical edge. *Administrative Theory & Praxis, 19,* 208–224.

Zanetti, L.A., & Carr, A. (2000). Contemporary pragmatism in public administration: Exploring the limitations of the "third productive reply." *Administration & Society, 32,* 433–452.

Zinn, H. (1999). *A people's history of the United States: 1492–present.* New York: HarperCollins.

Index

About the Author

Richard C. Box (D.P.A.) is a professor in the School of Public Administration, University of Nebraska at Omaha. He served for thirteen years as a land-use planner, department head, and city administrator in local governments in Oregon and California before completing his doctorate at the University of Southern California. His research focuses on democracy, citizen self-governance, and the application of critical thought in public administration.